UNDERSTANDING
MEDICINE

Dr Paul Whiteman

TEACH YOURSELF BOOKS

Cover photograph: J.C. REVY/SCIENCE PHOTO LIBRARY.
False-colour magnetic resonance image (MRI) of a whole
human body, a woman, taken in coronal (frontal) section.

Long-renowned as the authoritative source for self-guided learning – with more
than 30 million copies sold worldwide – the *Teach Yourself* series includes over
200 titles in the fields of languages, crafts, hobbies, sports, and other leisure
activities.

British Library Cataloguing in Publication Data
A catalogue for this title is available from the British Library.

Library of Congress Catalog Card Number: 96-68475

First published in UK 1996 by Hodder Headline Plc, 338 Euston Road, London
NW1 3BH

First published in US 1996 by NTC Publishing Group, 4255 West Touhy
Avenue, Lincolnwood (Chicago), Illinois 60646 – 1975 U.S.A.

Copyright © 1995 Paul Whiteman

In UK: All rights reserved. No part of this publication may be reproduced or
transmitted in any form or by any means, electronic or mechanical, including
photocopy, recording, or any information storage and retrieval system, without
permission in writing from the publisher or under licence from the Copyright
Licensing Agency Limited. Further details of such licences (for reprographic
reproduction) may be obtained from the Copyright Licensing Agency Limited,
of 90 Tottenham Court Road, London W1P 9HE.

In US: All rights reserved. No part of this book may be reproduced, stored in a
retrieval system, or transmitted in any form, or by any means, electronic,
mechanical, photocopying, or otherwise, without prior permission of NTC
Publishing Group.

Typeset by Transet Limited, Coventry, England.
Printed in England by Cox & Wyman Ltd, Reading, Berkshire.

Impression number	14	13	12	11	10	9	8	7	6	5	4	3	2
Year	1999		1998		1997		1996						

CONTENTS

PREFACE

This book aims to provide the reader who has no particular background in science or medicine with a reasonably in-depth understanding of some of the important fundamental principles, opinions and issues in modern orthodox medicine. It also provides a glimpse into the medical establishment and the ways doctors work. Teachers and other professionals who are not medically qualified but work in areas impinging on medical science and human biology, and possibly preclinical medical students, may find parts useful. Emphasis is mainly on some of the major medical problems in countries like the UK. Medical science continues to advance rapidly and medical practices, opinions and services are at present in a state of considerable flux. *Understanding Medicine* conveys merely a snapshot in time. This book is not meant to be a home doctor. It should *not* be used to make a diagnosis, offer clinical advice or suggest a treatment.

I thank Janet Whiteman, my wife, for tremendous support and encouragement, for ideas and helpful discussions and for reading manuscripts and proofs.

Paul Whiteman

1

INTRODUCTION

Medicine now

Most people in developed countries can expect to live beyond 70 years. The major causes of death in middle age are coronary artery disease and cancer. The risk of premature death from these diseases can often be reduced by relatively simple preventive measures; the problem is how to encourage those most at risk to use the available services and to make the necessary lifestyle changes. The proportion of elderly people in the population is rising, bringing new social, medical and economic challenges.

Most people with serious illness turn to conventional medicine, which generally offers the best hope of cure or relief. Modern medicine must by its very nature be in a state of change, adapting to new ideas and practices and striving to meet the changing needs and demands of society. Medical science, technology and opinion continues to evolve rapidly. The advances provide many options for patient care, but costs are escalating and choices cannot always be based on clinical need alone. The health services are now having to focus more coherently on the most important medical and social issues and to develop clearer strategies for the future. The greater and sometimes unrealistic expectations of patients often cannot be met in practice. There is also the spectre of ever increasing litigation and its effect on costs.

Practising doctors primarily make clinical management decisions on clinical grounds, but increasingly they are having to take costs into account and the services they may wish to offer their patients may not always be in their gift. People may now wish to have more open and more meaningful discussions with their doctors when negotiating options for the management of their health problems in an increasingly money-oriented health market.

About this book

This book aims to help the reader develop an understanding of some of the important principles, issues and opinions in modern orthodox medicine and to provide an insight into the ways doctors think and work. It will *not* teach you how to practise medicine, neither should it be used to make a diagnosis, offer clinical advice or suggest a treatment.

In order to achieve the main aim of the book in less than 250 pages the author has been ruthlessly selective in the choice of topics. Emphasis is mainly on major medical issues in countries like the UK. The major health problems and priorities in underdeveloped and tropical countries are quite different and would require a different book to do them justice. To enable the lay person to develop their understanding as they progress through this book the presentation and the arrangement of subject matter is of necessity unconventional.

Chapters two and three introduce human biology and disease and provide the basis for the rest of the book.

The medical establishment

Doctors have overall and ultimate responsibility for the clinical management of patients under their care. They decide what the disease is and its cause (**diagnosis**), determine the likely course of the illness and the clinical prospects for the patient (**prognosis**) and decide upon and prescribe the appropriate treatment.

The medical degree course lasts five or six years, three of which are clinical years involving work with patients. In the UK, most medical students receive Bachelor of Medicine and Bachelor of Surgery degrees (MB, BS or equivalent) when they pass their final examinations at the end of the course. They may then use the title 'Dr' but they are not licensed to practise medicine. To become a fully-registered medical practitioner (General Medical Council registration) entitled to practise independently as a medical doctor the new graduate must first satisfactorily complete one year working in hospital as a houseman (intern). This is an intensive and usually gruelling residential year in which fledgling doctors consolidate their skills in patient care and responsibility under the guidance of more senior doctors.

For a career in general (family) practice a doctor must now also have an additional three years of vocational experience in suitable hospital and general practice training posts. For those bent on a career in hospital medicine the training is longer and the outcome less certain. The term junior hospital doctor refers to those in the various hospital training grades (e.g. senior house officers, registrars).

Consultants are senior hospital doctors, the archetypal specialists. The great majority are consultant physicians or consultant surgeons. The standards required of consultants in the National Health Service are high and there is fierce competition for relatively few jobs, especially in the teaching hospitals (those training medical students). Virtually every consultant will have a higher medical qualification from the relevant specialist college (e.g. Membership of the Royal College of Physicians – MRCP, Fellowship of the Royal College of Surgeons – FRCS). Doctors with appropriate experience and qualifications can register as specialists without a consultant appointment.

Physicians may specialise in **general medicine** (the commonest), **paediatrics** (children), **geriatrics** (the elderly), **chest medicine**, **dermatology** (skin), **venereology** (sexually-transmitted diseases), **rheumatology**, **oncology** (cancer), **neurology** (nervous system) and **cardiology** (heart). Later chapters mention the surgical specialities and other specialist hospital posts held by doctors. There are many areas outside mainstream medicine in which medical doctors play an important role, such as occupational health, public health, the pharmaceutical industry, and government and its agencies.

Established practitioners and specialists keep abreast of medical practice by reading professional journals and attending post-graduate courses. In the UK, this continuing medical education has lacked coordination, and keeping up-to-date has been largely a matter of self-regulation by the individual doctor. Future arrangements for professional accreditation will probably address these shortfalls.

In some countries doctors qualify with a doctor of medicine degree (e.g. MD). In the UK, the MD or DM is a post-graduate degree awarded to medical practitioners for medical research. Most non-medical doctors have a Doctor of Philosophy degree (PhD), also for research. Just to add to the confusion, surgeons in the UK traditionally use the title 'Mr', even though they are entitled to use 'Dr'. In this book the term doctor refers to any conventionally qualified medical practitioner.

— Basic medical services in the UK —

Patient care in the National Health Service (NHS) is broadly divided into primary, secondary and tertiary care. The initial point of contact for the patient is at the primary care level. The primary health care team includes the general practitioners and associated general practice staff. All UK residents have the right to register with an NHS general practitioner. Secondary care involves hospital-based specialist diagnosis and treatment. Apart from certain emergency services and genito-urinary medicine clinics (for sexually transmitted diseases), the patient does not normally have direct access to NHS secondary care facilities unless referred by the general practitioner, who essentially acts as a gate-keeper between primary and secondary care. This protects the patient from the disadvantages of unnecessary exposure to hospitals, ensures referral to the most appropriate specialist and allows efficient use of resources. The primary health care team also provides health education and disease prevention services.

Tertiary care is very specialised treatment available only in a few centres (e.g. heart surgery, radiotherapy); the patient is referred by a hospital specialist.

When opting for private hospital medicine it is still advisable to obtain advice from a general practitioner, and specialists usually expect to receive a letter of referral. The NHS generally provides all the essential medical services required for the seriously ill. It also trains doctors and nurses. The private sector can often offer a quicker and more convenient service for one-off non-emergency treatments, but it does not in general cater well for the chronically sick nor for emergency medicine and surgery. In some areas a closer link between the NHS and private sector facilities has led to mutual benefits.

Changes in the financing of the NHS now allow many general practitioners to make selective purchases of secondary care for their patients and to set contract standards. Purchasing and budgets are geared to provide the most appropriate services to meet identified medical needs and priorities in the population. In practice this will occasionally mean that individual patients will not always get all the services they expect. Doctors will continue to operate in the best clinical interests of their patients but their ability to manoeuvre may become increasingly influenced by economic considerations. Patients can quite reasonably expect their doctors to discuss with them the clinical options available for the management of their condition and also any financial constraints that limit the choice. The customer may need to ask more questions than before, and be prepared to negotiate and, if necessary, seek advice elsewhere.

2
THE BODY

Form and function

Traditionally, study of the human body is divided into separate subjects, such as anatomy, physiology and biochemistry, each with its own specialists, particular laboratory techniques and textbooks. **Anatomy** is concerned with form and structure, **physiology** with function, and **biochemistry** with chemical processes. These subjects are closely interrelated and in this book they will be integrated as far as possible. Form and function can be considered from the visible anatomical level down to the smallest parts of matter, atoms and molecules. The following sections expand on this theme and introduce basic terms and concepts.

Some basic chemistry

A knowledge of chemistry is essential for a thorough understanding of many aspects of modern medicine. Fortunately, a little knowledge will take us quite a long way.

We, and all the substances around us, whether gas, liquid or solid, are composed of **atoms**, the smallest individual units of matter. The types and the arrangements of atoms in a material determine its properties. Although there are many types, here we need only consider **hydrogen**, **oxygen**, **nitrogen** and **carbon** atoms. By convention they are represented by the symbols **H**, **O**, **N** and **C** respectively. These atoms do not normally remain in a free single state but interact to form joined-up groups of atoms called **molecules**. Figure 2.1 depicts the

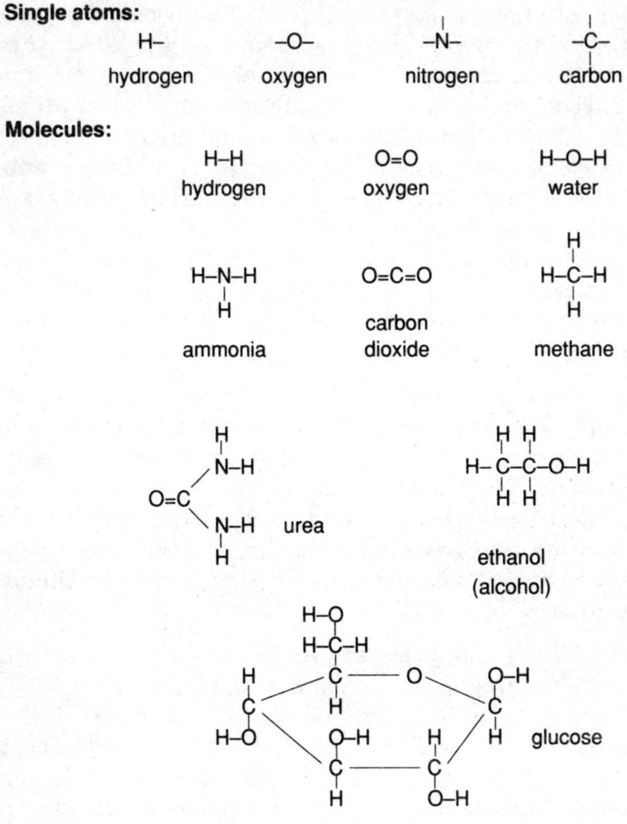

Single atoms:

H–	–O–	–N̶–	–C̶–
hydrogen	oxygen	nitrogen	carbon

Molecules:

H–H   O=O   H–O–H
hydrogen   oxygen   water

H–N–H   O=C=O   methane
   |
   H
ammonia   carbon
             dioxide

urea

ethanol
(alcohol)

glucose

Figure 2.1 Atoms and molecules

molecules of some well known substances. Note how the atoms are linked together. Hydrogen, which is the simplest and smallest atom, has only one link with which to form electronic bonds with links on other atoms. Oxygen, nitrogen and carbon atoms respectively typically have two, three and four links available for bonding. Thus, the molecular formulae for hydrogen, water, ammonia and methane (marsh gas) are conventionally written as H_2, H_2O, NH_3 and CH_4 respectively (see figure 2.1). Molecules are the smallest particles that retain the characteristics of the substance, such as the smell of ammonia and the flammability of methane. Most things around us are composed of complex mixtures of molecules and have correspondingly more complicated properties.

A substance composed of just one type of atom is called an **element** and has the same chemical name as the atom. For example, in their pure forms the substances we call iron, sulphur and carbon contain only iron, sulphur and carbon atoms respectively. Charcoal, graphite and diamond are also forms of the element carbon; the very different properties of these substances are due entirely to the way the carbon atoms are arranged. The gases hydrogen, oxygen and nitrogen are also elements; their molecules consist of two like atoms joined together. Carbon dioxide, a gas formed in the body and expelled through the lungs, is not an element because its molecules contain two different types of atom, oxygen and carbon.

The carbon atom is remarkable. It is the basis of the vast array of simple and complex molecules that form living things. It can combine with other carbon atoms to form chains or rings and with different types such as hydrogen, oxygen and nitrogen. Sugars and fats are formed from combinations of carbon, hydrogen and oxygen atoms. In the body these substances may be stored, become part of a structure or be chemically burnt to provide energy.

The molecule of the simple sugar **glucose** contains six carbon atoms, twelve hydrogen atoms and six oxygen atoms; its chemical formula can therefore be written as $C_6H_{12}O_6$. The **structural formula** (see figure 2.1, page 7) shows how these atoms are linked together. In the body, six molecules of oxygen (O_2) can release the chemical energy from one molecule of glucose. The series of chemical reactions involved ultimately convert the oxygen and glucose into carbon dioxide (CO_2) and water (H_2O). The following chemical equation summarises the overall process.

$$C_6H_{12}O_6 \ + \ 6\,O_2 \ = \ 6\,CO_2 \ + 6\,H_2O \ + \ \text{energy}$$

glucose   oxygen   carbon   water
dioxide

The function of the lungs is to take in the oxygen required from the air and to expel excess carbon dioxide.

Proteins consist of chains of individual molecular structures called **amino acids**, of which there are some twenty different types; examples are shown in figure 2.2. Some proteins form

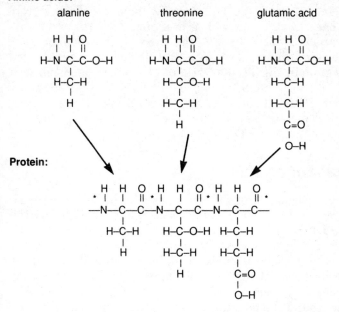

Figure 2.2 Amino acids and protein
Amino acids contain a -NH₂ (amino) group and an acidic -CO.OH (carboxyl) group. During protein synthesis the amino group on one amino acid reacts with the carboxyl group on another to form a peptide bond (*). A water molecule is lost in the reaction.

part of the structure of the body and others have very special functions, such as the **enzymes** which facilitate specific chemical changes. For instance, a series of enzymes convert glucose and oxygen into carbon dioxide and water. All amino acids, and therefore all proteins, contain carbon, hydrogen, oxygen and nitrogen (two amino acids also contain a sulphur atom). Amino-acid nitrogen in excess of requirements is incorporated, by chemical processes in the liver, into a simple non-toxic substance called **urea** (see figure 2.1) which readily passes through the kidneys into the urine.

Metabolism is an overall term used to describe all the chemical processes in a living thing or all the chemical processes affecting a particular substance in a living thing (e.g. the body's metabolism, the metabolism of glucose). Two particular states of metabolism are **anabolism** and **catabolism**. Anabolism refers to the building of complex molecules from simple ones, such as protein from amino acids (think of anabolic steroids). Catabolism is the process in which complex molecules are broken down into simpler ones (e.g. breakdown of body protein during starvation). Normal metabolism is a balance of many anabolic and catabolic activities. Virtually every one of the thousands of individual chemical reactions involved in metabolism requires the assistance of an individual purpose-made highly specific enzyme.

More about protein

There are thousands of different proteins in the body, each playing a special role in keeping us alive and well. The particularity of their role, or function, is determined entirely by their structure and form. Although we eat proteins from a variety of sources, such as plants and other animals, we do not incorporate these as such. In the stomach and bowel they are broken down into component amino acids which are then distributed around the body to be used as building blocks for the manufacture of our own particular brands of proteins. In fact, our **genes** define precisely how the amino acids are to be linked together.

Figure 2.2 (page 9) illustrates part of a protein chain containing the amino acids alanine, threonine and glutamic acid. Note how they are linked together by special bonds between carbon and nitrogen atoms (the **peptide bond**). A protein molecule comprises rows of hundreds of amino acids joined together in this way. As there are 20 different amino acids the possibility for structural individuality is astronomical. The amino acids have different properties and their arrangement in the chain confers particular characteristics to the protein; some parts like to stay in contact with their watery surroundings, others prefer not to, and some parts have particular types of electrical charge causing attraction and repulsion.

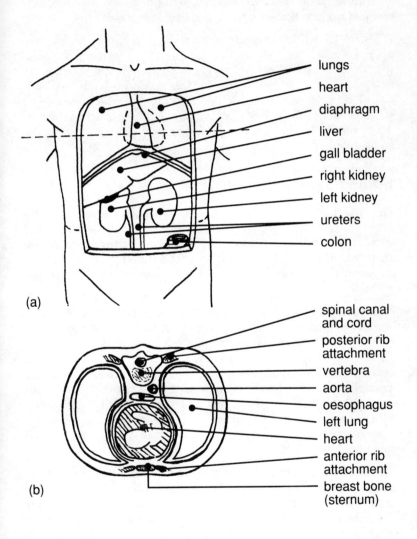

Figure 2.3 The thoracic and abdominal cavities
(**a**) The front wall of the trunk has been removed to show some of the internal organs. The heart is largely obscured by the lungs. The abdominal cavity lies below the diaphragm. Stomach and bowels are removed to show the kidneys. Cut end of the lower colon is indicated.
(**b**) Horizontal section through the chest at the level indicated by broken line in (a).

Therefore many proteins do not remain as extended chains but fold up into complex three dimensional structures.

It is the particular contour of physical and chemical features on the surface of the protein that confers its uniqueness of function, its **specificity**. Two types of protein that display an extreme degree of specificity are the **enzymes** and **antibodies**. They interact with, and do things to, other molecular structures, but only those having particular characteristics. In other words they recognise specific molecules or parts of molecules, just as a lock recognises a key.

Some basic anatomy

The internal organs performing the essential house-keeping functions are situated in the two large compartments of the trunk, the **thoracic cavity** in the chest (**thorax**) and the **abdominal cavity** below it. Figure 2.3 illustrates some of the anatomical relationships (for clarity several structures are omitted).

The two lungs occupy most of the thoracic cavity and the heart lies at its centre. They are protected by the bony rib cage which provides rigidity to the chest wall and assists breathing. Below them is the **diaphragm**, a muscular partition separating the two compartments. When its muscles shorten (**contract**) it is drawn downwards, forcing the lungs to expand and take in air. Due to their elasticity the lungs shrink back as the diaphragm relaxes and air is expelled. Normal quiet breathing is due mainly to the up and down movements of the diaphragm.

The abdominal cavity lies below the diaphragm and contains many organs. The liver is the largest, occupying the right upper region. The two kidneys lie at the back of the cavity on either side. The guts, that is the stomach and intestines (bowels), occupy most of the remaining space and are part of the system of passages, known as the **digestive tract** or **alimentary canal**, responsible for the transit and processing of food. They move around more and change shape according to needs.

Attributes, functions and events relating to the heart, lungs, liver, kidneys and stomach respectively are described by the adjectives **cardiac**, **pulmonary**, **hepatic**, **renal** and **gastric** (e.g. cardiac arrest, renal failure).

The backbone (**vertebral** or **spinal column**) is the most primordial structure of the skeleton, and its presence, or a rudimentary form of it, is the primary characteristic of one of the great subdivisions of the animal kingdom, the **chordates**, to which of course we belong. The vertebral column consists of a series of individual bones called **vertebrae** (singular, vertebra) separated from each other by **intervertebral discs**. In humans the top seven form the bones of the neck (**cervical vertebrae**), the next twelve are the **thoracic vertebrae** at the back of the chest, supporting the ribs, and beneath them are the five **lumbar vertebrae** in the lower back. The stiffness of the spine provides support to the body but its joints and muscles also allow a degree of flexibility and movement. The vertebral column and the activity of its associated muscles maintain and control posture.

The top cervical vertebra supports the skull. Below the fifth (lowest) lumbar vertebra the bones of the spine are fused together and attached to the large bones of the pelvis.

The skull and the vertebral column provide bony protection for the most intricate and vulnerable parts of the nervous system, the brain and its extension, the **spinal cord**. The latter passes through a hole at the bottom of the skull into the **spinal canal**, a tunnel running down through the vertebral column behind the main bodies of the bones and their interconnecting discs. On both sides nerves arise from the spinal cord and pass through small holes between the vertebrae to supply the trunk and limbs. Note the different meanings of the terms spinal (or vertebral) **column**, spinal **canal** and spinal **cord**.

Certain terms describing spatial orientation are used frequently in anatomy and medicine. **Anterior**, **posterior**, **superior** and **inferior** refer to positions in front, behind, above and below respectively. There are some pairs of words which more or less mean inner and outer. They are: **central** and **peripheral**, **medial** and **lateral** (towards the middle and side respectively), and **proximal** and **distal** (nearest and farthest from the centre respectively).

There are several levels of organisation between molecules and man. Important ones are **cells**, **tissues**, **organs** and **systems**.

Cells and tissues

What are cells?

The human body is a society of around ten million million individual cells, the smallest units capable of functioning independently as living things. To ensure our continuing health the activities and behaviour of the member cells must be strictly channelled and controlled.

Animals consisting of just one cell, a group known as **protozoa**, like the tiny amoeba found in ponds, display all the characteristics of living things. They interact with their environment, sensing and moving about, seeking out favourable conditions for survival. They take in nutrients, process and utilise them according to needs, such as growth and maintenance, and expel waste materials. The energy required to power these activities comes from the chemical breakdown, within the cell, of food fuels. They also reproduce themselves, ensuring perpetuation of the species.

In multicellular animals, like us, different groups of cells become specialised to carry out particular functions more effectively. This specialisation may involve extreme exaggeration of one characteristic, such as movement in muscle cells and the transmission of electrical messages in nerve cells (**neurons**). Other activities may be suppressed; neurons are unable to reproduce themselves to replace damaged ones. Most cells retain the ability to carry out basic house-keeping functions such as utilising nutrients, expelling waste and generating the energy needed to do their work.

Cells may be the smallest independent units of life but they are far from simple. The three major components of a cell are the **cytoplasm**, **cell membrane** and **nucleus** (see figure 2.4). Cytoplasm is like a highly organized soup. It contains many

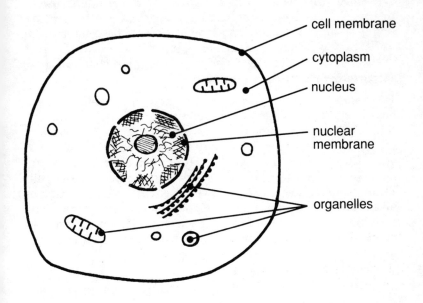

Figure 2.4 The cell

complex structures, collectively known as organelles, different types having different functions. Most of the cell's house-keeping activities take place in the cytoplasm.

The cell membrane surrounding the cytoplasm is the point of contact with the outside world. It helps maintain a controlled internal environment by selectively taking in and expelling materials. Gases pass across the membrane through minute pores in its molecular structure. The concentration of oxygen molecules inside the cell tends to be low because oxygen atoms are constantly being incorporated into chemical reactions. Oxygen dissolved in the fluid outside the cell is usually present at higher concentrations so that more oxygen molecules pass in than out. Due to metabolism carbon dioxide molecules accumulate inside the cell and effect a net flow outwards across the membrane.

The **nucleus** is a roughly spherical compartment within the cytoplasm from which it is separated by the **nuclear membrane**. The nucleus is the cell's management centre, controlling growth, the amount and type of work to be done and the utilisation of resources. Efficient communication with the rest of the cell is achieved by a two-way passage of chemical messages across the nuclear membrane.

The data required to operate the cell, and for reproduction, are held in structures called **chromosomes**. The nuclei of human cells contain 46 chromosomes, two matching sets of 23. One set holds the information inherited from the father and the other that from the mother. The chromosomes contain genetic information for the whole body, not just for one type of cell. Throughout development, from the early embryo consisting of just a few cells to the final adult human form, the missions, activities and fates of different groups of cells are determined by modifying access to particular parts of the data base.

Each chromosome consists of various specialised proteins and one very long molecular structure known as **DNA** (deoxyribonucleic acid), the famous **double helix**. DNA is the data base of the cell. It contains the information needed for the manufacture of proteins, and for reproduction.

Genes and proteins

A **gene** is a discrete portion of DNA holding the data required for the manufacture (**synthesis**) of one specific protein chain. Each DNA molecule, and therefore each chromosome, contains thousands of such genes.

Inactive DNA exists in the chromosome as tightly bunched coiled coils. When protein synthesis is required the coils unravel and the relevant part of the DNA molecule is made available for reading. DNA consists of two extremely long molecules held closely together, rather like a two-stranded twine (double helix). Each strand can be likened to a row of millions of beads, of which there are just four different types. Each bead represents a chemical subunit, a molecular structure,

Nucleus:

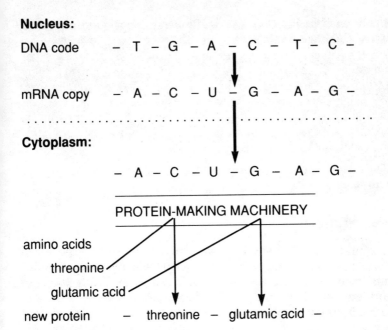

Figure 2.5   How DNA determines protein structure (refer to text)

known as a base. By convention the chemical names of the different types of base are abbreviated to **A** (adenine), **T** (thymine), **G** (guanine) and **C** (cytosine). When new protein is needed the bases on the relevant gene are *read*, in one direction. Each of the 20 amino acids is represented by particular sequences of three bases. For example, the amino acids threonine and glutamic acid have the DNA codes TGA and CTC respectively. These three-base sequences are known as **codons** or **triplet**s. They are the basis of the **genetic code**.

Figure 2.5 illustrates how DNA conveys its message for protein synthesis. In double-stranded DNA, **A**s on one strand stick to **T**s on the other, and similarly **G**s stick to **C**s. In fact the two strands are exactly complementary. When protein synthesis is required they separate and another molecule called **RNA** (ribonucleic acid), very similar to DNA, is built alongside the protein-coding strand. The RNA so formed also has a complementary structure, except that one of the bases is different; **U** (uridine) replaces **T**, but retains the affinity for **A**. When completed the RNA molecule contains its own code for the manufacture of one particular protein and it takes the message to specialised organelles in the cytoplasm where amino acids are assembled into protein. This particular form of RNA is known as **messenger RNA** (or mRNA). Conventionally, the codons for amino acids are written in terms of mRNA sequences, rather than DNA sequences; thus the codon for threonine becomes ACU.

The nucleus regulates cellular activity by controlling protein synthesis.

Reproduction

Due to a short life span, or wear and tear, some specialised cells in the body require continual replacement with new ones. Important examples are blood cells and those lining the skin and gut. A small number of less specialised predecessors called **stem cells** oblige by reproducing. First they make a complete replica of their DNA, giving rise to two complete sets of chromosomes. Then the nucleus divides into two, each half taking one complete set (i.e. 46 chromosomes). Finally, the cytoplasm between the nuclei separates to produce two new daughter cells. But they may have different destinies. One transforms into the replacement specialised cell, a process called **differentiation**, but the other may retain the properties of an undifferentiated stem cell, thus providing a continuing source of replenishment.

At the stage of DNA replication the two original strands separate and both are copied, so that each daughter cell gets a copy of the DNA that codes for protein and a copy of the complementary DNA strand. This method of cell reproduction, in which the daughter nuclei contain the same number of chromosomes as the parent nucleus, is known as **mitosis**.

Sexual reproduction is different, in several ways. It concerns only the cells of the **gonads**, the ovaries and testicles, and the female egg cells (**ova**) and male **sperm** cells arising respectively from them. At an early stage the cells contain 46 chromosomes, just like the other cells of the body. Then, within the same cell, the maternal and paternal chromosomes line up and some genetic material is exchanged between the matching pairs. Subsequent cell divisions give rise to ova and sperms with just one set of 23 chromosomes each. If mating is successful, a sperm unites with an ovum to produce a new cell (the **zygote**) with a nucleus containing a complete set of 46 chromosomes (fertilisation, conception). The process allows considerable variation in genetic stock which may through natural selection provide evolutionary advantage.

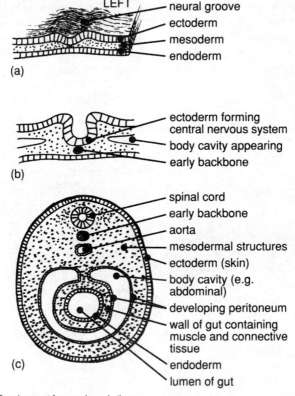

Figure 2.6 Development from embryonic tissues
(a) Cross-section through a three week embryo (just over 1 mm long). It shows the three embryonic tissue layers from which all parts develop. The neural groove is the beginning of the nervous system.
(b) Cross-section at a later stage.
(c) A very diagrammatic cross-section at an even later stage of development. It shows how the embryonic tissues form and separate into the major structures and compartments of the body. The endoderm becomes the layer of cells lining the inside of the gut. The mesoderm forms muscle, bone, cartilage, heart and blood vessels. The ectoderm forms skin and nervous system.

Tissues

The zygote is the first cell of the developing human being. Subsequent cell divisions (by mitosis) lead to an increasing degree of specialisation in particular groups of cells. When the zygote first divides, the daughter cells have the potential to form complete human beings, and occasionally they do so by forming identical twins. After a few divisions specialisation occurs in different parts of the growing cell colony. Within three weeks of conception three distinct layers of cells are present from which all parts of the embryo will develop. Some of the processes involved are illustrated in a very diagrammatic form in figure 2.6. Strictly, the developing human is called an **embryo** for the first two months after conception and a **fetus**

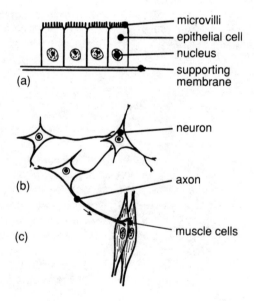

(a)
microvilli
epithelial cell
nucleus
supporting membrane

(b)
neuron
axon

(c)
muscle cells

Figure 2.7 Examples of tissues
(a) Typical of epithelium lining the small bowel.
The microvilli increase the area for absorption of nutrients.
(b) A simple network of nerve cells (neurons).
(c) An axon (nerve fibre) from a neuron supplies motor signals to muscle cells. Muscle tissue consists of complex bundles of muscle cells.

(or foetus) thereafter until birth.

The term **tissue** usually refers to a group of cells with similar form and function. The three embryonic tissues referred to above give rise to more distinct tissues which, once formed, cannot convert into other types. For instance, the primitive **ectoderm** differentiates into nervous tissue and the outer layer of the skin (**epidermis**), but once formed skin cells cannot convert to nerve cells, nor vice versa.

As shown in figure 2.6, all three primitive tissues (**ectoderm**, **endoderm** and **mesoderm**) can produce membranes, sheets of cells joined closely together to provide a protective or limiting lining or boundary. The term **epithelium** is applied to this kind of tissue; there are several distinct types with different functions. One type of membrane arising from mesoderm lines the insides of the major cavities of the trunk. In the abdomen this membrane is the **peritoneum**. It covers some of the abdominal organs and is continuous with a layer lining the inside of the body wall (see figure 2.6). Normally there is no space between the inner and outer layers, just a little lubricating fluid to allow the surfaces to glide smoothly over each other. A similar membrane covers the heart and lungs in the thoracic cavity where it is called the **pericardium** and **pleura** respectively.

Examples of a few tissues and their particular types of cell are shown in figure 2.7. Note how the epithelial cells lining the inside of the small bowel have numerous projections to increase the area available for absorption of nutrients and how neurons form communication networks through extensions of the cell body. There are different types of muscle cell. Those forming the muscle tissue attached to the skeleton and responsible for movement (e.g. walking) under conscious control are different to those that act automatically in internal structures such as the heart and within the walls of the blood vessels and the gut.

The term tissue can be confusing. The function of a tissue is generally determined by one type of cell, but there may be others present in a supporting role. **Connective tissues** support and protect the other tissues and organs and fill in spaces. In some of these the main function is provided by structures situated outside the cells, such as tough protein fibres (e.g. collagen) that provide mechanical strength. Examples of connective tissues are bone, cartilage, the tissues forming tendons or ligaments, and **adipose tissue** which contains cells laden with fat (fat cells – the fat storage system).

Obviously, very precise mechanisms must operate in the tissues, and especially in developing tissues, to ensure that cells muster in the correct location and in the right number. Special molecules on the cell surface are involved in recognition processes and local chemical messages are important in controlling cell growth and reproduction. Given the phenomenal number and complexity of cellular changes occurring in the embryo, it is not surprising that many chemicals, including some drugs, can interfere with normal development.

Tissue fluids

Water accounts for more than half the weight of a non-obese man, and most of it is inside the cells. The rest is in the blood plasma and the fluid surrounding the cells, the **interstitial fluid**. The latter represents the equivalent of the amoeba's pond. The cells of the body need to bathe in fluid in order to take up nutrients and oxygen, expel waste and exchange chemical messages. The composition of interstitial fluid must be carefully controlled to prevent cellular damage. This function is delegated to particular organs, such as the kidney (see page 40). At this point we shall just consider briefly the distribution of water and some important mineral salts.

Sodium chloride is better known as common salt; it is also the main mineral salt in the interstitial fluid bathing the cells. When dissolved in water its constituent sodium and chlorine atoms separate and gain electrical charges, the sodium atoms become positively charged and the chlorine atoms negatively charged. Electrically charged atoms are called **ions**. The main positive mineral ion inside the cell is **potassium** (similar to sodium but the atom is bigger). Special pumps (specific proteins) in the cell membrane maintain the higher potassium and lower sodium ion concentrations in the cell. Electrical activities in cell membranes, such as the transmission of nerve messages, are due to changes in the distribution of ions.

Unlike many of the substances dissolved in it, water moves freely across most human cell membranes. It is drawn towards the compartment containing the highest concentration of dissolved particles (the sum of all the molecules and ions). This process is called **osmosis**, which may be defined as the tendency of water in a less concentrated solution to pass through a membrane selectively permeable to water into a more concentrated solution until both are of the same concentration. Under normal circumstances the **osmotic pressure**, the force tending to move water across, is similar in the fluids inside and outside the cell, so there are only small changes in the water content and volume of the cell. Sodium and chloride ions account for about three-quarters of the osmotic pressure of the interstitial fluid; many other substances contribute to the remainder.

A solution containing nine grams of pure sodium chloride per litre of water has an osmotic pressure similar to that of interstitial fluid. It is known as **isotonic** or **normal saline** and, after sterilisation, is used frequently in clinical practice (e.g. to bathe damaged tissues, as a vehicle for injection, for body fluid replacement).

Blood

Blood comprises **red cells**, **white cells** and **platelets** suspended in a protein-rich liquid called **plasma**. After birth, blood cell manufacture takes place in the marrow cavities of the bones. In the adult this activity is normally restricted to particular bones such as the breastbone, ribs, vertebrae and the upper parts of the pelvic bone.

Red cells account for more than 99 per cent of the cells in blood and are so abundant they occupy nearly half its volume. They are disc shaped, have lost their nuclei and are extremely specialised. Their major function is to transport oxygen. Red cells are laden, to one-third of their weight, with a red oxygen-carrying substance called **haemoglobin**, which consists of an iron-containing component (haem) and protein (globin). The white cells are a mixed group of cells particularly involved in the fight against infection. The bloodstream transports them to the battlefields.

Platelets are small specialised fragments of cytoplasm surrounded by a membrane. They play a vital role in the repair and maintenance of blood vessel walls by sticking to damaged areas and plugging small breaches. They also participate in the clotting of blood.

Apart from its high protein concentration, plasma is very similar to interstitial fluid. The most abundant protein dissolved in plasma is **albumin** which facilitates water flow between plasma and the interstitial fluid in the tissues. Other plasma proteins are the **globulins**, a group which includes the antibodies, and **fibrinogen** which is essential for clot formation.

When blood is placed in a glass vessel the fibrinogen changes from its soluble (dissolved) form into an insoluble polymer called **fibrin**. The latter enmeshes the blood cells in a fibrous network which eventually contracts to form a clot. The fluid left on the outside is **serum**, which is plasma without the fibrinogen.

There is a constant need to repair even the smallest amount of damage in blood vessel walls to prevent bleeding and ensure smooth blood flow. The role of the platelets has been mentioned. When damage to the vessel wall is more extensive the platelets and injured tissues involved emit chemical messages which activate clot formation in the vicinity. The clotting mechanism involves a number of specialised plasma proteins which act sequentially upon each other until eventually fibrinogen is converted to fibrin. The developing clot cements the platelet plug firmly to the damaged wall.

This highly effective plumbing repair system must be carefully regulated to prevent its activities extending beyond the damaged area. The internal surface of the healthy blood vessel does not favour clot formation. It emits chemicals that prevent platelets sticking and fibrin clots forming. Activation of another plasma protein system produces **plasmin** which dismantles unwanted local fibrin after the repair. Yet another system regulates plasmin activity.

Defects in these systems cause a variety of clinical disorders characterised by abnormal bleeding or clotting.

—— The heart and the circulation ——

The circulatory system

In order to function effectively, tissues require a continuous supply of oxygen and nutrients and efficient removal of their waste products. The circulation of the blood provides the vehicle for the transport of these substances between pick-up and delivery points. It also rapidly distributes the special chemical messengers (**hormones**) that control and co-ordinate metabolic activities in different parts of the body.

A continuous oxygen supply is particularly important. Without it vital brain cells rapidly die. When blood passes through the lungs, oxygen in the inhaled air is extracted and fixed onto haemoglobin in the red cells. The heart pumps the oxygen-rich (**oxygenated**) blood to the tissues (e.g. brain, muscle), where local conditions encourage haemoglobin to release its oxygen.

The delivery of oxygenated blood to the tissues is achieved by means of a double circulation, known variously as the **circulatory system** or the **blood vascular system**.

The double circulation is easily understood by visualising a continuous tube looped in a figure-of-eight arrangement. In the top loop, blood flows through the lungs absorbing oxygen; this is the **pulmonary circulation**. In the other loop, blood passes through the rest of the body, giving up its oxygen to the tissues; this is the **systemic circulation**.

The adult vascular system contains about five litres of blood which always circulates in one direction.

The heart

The heart is the pump at the centre of the system, where the loops of the double circulation cross over (see figure 2.8). It consists of two separate pumping units, sometimes called the left and right hearts because of their anatomical relationship. Each unit comprises a chamber which receives incoming blood (**atrium**), a chamber with a very muscular wall which pumps

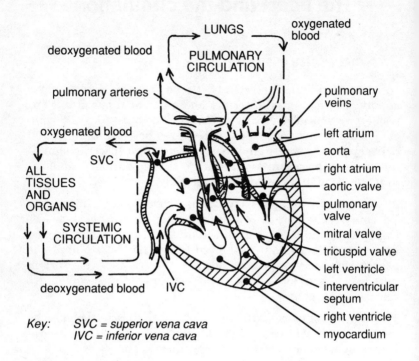

LUNGS — oxygenated blood

PULMONARY CIRCULATION

deoxygenated blood

pulmonary arteries

oxygenated blood

SVC

ALL TISSUES AND ORGANS

SYSTEMIC CIRCULATION

deoxygenated blood   IVC

pulmonary veins

left atrium

aorta

right atrium

aortic valve

pulmonary valve

mitral valve

tricuspid valve

left ventricle

interventricular septum

right ventricle

myocardium

Key: SVC = superior vena cava
        IVC = inferior vena cava

Figure 2.8   The heart and the double circulation

blood into the arteries (**ventricle**), and a set of valves to ensure that blood flows only in one direction.

The course of the circulatory system can now be reviewed in more detail (see figure 2.8). Oxygenated blood from the lungs returns to the heart via the pulmonary veins and is collected into the **left atrium**. The heart relaxes and the **mitral valve** opens, allowing blood to pass from the left atrium to the **left ventricle**. The latter contracts, forcing the mitral valve to close, and ejects its contents through the **aortic valve** into the **aorta**, the great artery transporting oxygenated blood to the body.

Oxygen-depleted (**deoxygenated**) blood from the tissues returns to the heart via the **superior** and **inferior venae**

cavae (singular, vena cava), the great veins draining the upper and lower body respectively, and is collected into the **right atrium**. From here it flows across the **tricuspid valve** into the **right ventricle** which, in turn, pumps the blood through the **pulmonary valve** into the **pulmonary arteries**. Thus, blood returns to the lungs to be re-oxygenated and the cycle starts again.

It is the same volume of blood that flows continuously round the vascular system; the left and right ventricles need to pump out similar amounts at each stroke, and at the same time. Special mechanisms are present to regulate and coordinate pump action according to requirements.

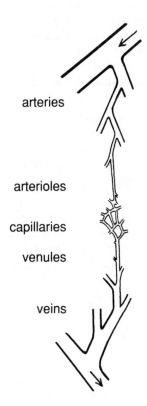

arteries

arterioles

capillaries

venules

veins

Figure 2.9 Blood vessels

Capillaries, arteries and veins

The purpose of the heart, arteries and veins is to get blood to and from the **capillaries**, the microscopic vessels which form vast networks (**capillary beds**) in the tissues (see figure 2.9). The internal bore of the capillary is so narrow that blood cells squeeze through in single file! The capillary wall consists of a single layer of cells called the **endothelium** (the name given to epithelium lining blood vessels) across which water, gases and various soluble materials can be exchanged between blood and tissue. Most blood cells, platelets and very large molecules, such as plasma proteins, stay within the blood vascular system.

The different types of vessel linked together to provide a passage for the blood are shown in figure 2.9. The endothelium of the capillaries extends into the arteries and veins so that it forms a continuous lining to the channel (or **lumen**). Unlike the capillaries, the other vessels have additional layers in their walls, and they do not allow exchange of substances with surrounding tissues.

The three layers of the arterial wall are: outermost, a tough fibrous and elastic coat (**tunica adventitia**), a middle layer consisting of muscle and elastic fibres (**tunica media**), and the innermost layer with the endothelium (**tunica intima**) (see figure 3.1 on page 56).

The larger arteries have a higher proportion of elastic fibre in the tunica media, so that they can expand to accommodate the blood ejected under pressure from the left ventricle and then continue to release it into the peripheral circulation after the aortic valve has closed. Muscle fibres dominate the walls of the smallest arterial vessels, which, by reducing (constricting) or increasing (dilating) the bore of the lumen, regulate blood flow and pressure.

The vein wall also possesses three layers but is much thinner, and the lumen is more capacious, offering a low resistance path to the large volume of blood returning to the heart at low pressure. The venous system acts as a reservoir; it contains two-thirds of the blood volume. Unlike arteries, many of the systemic veins (but not the pulmonary veins) have valves to prevent backflow.

Heart beats and pulses

Typically, in an adult at rest, the heart beats (pumps) about 70 times per minute (**heart rate**) and ejects about 70 millilitres (ml) of blood from the left ventricle at each beat (**stroke volume**). This gives a cardiac output of about five litres per minute. So, it takes only a minute for each ventricle to expel the total blood volume.

Blood ejected from the left ventricle travels rapidly in a wave through the large elastic arteries towards the periphery. This can be easily felt as a pulse at the wrist (**radial artery**), groin (**femoral artery**) and neck (**carotid artery**). Normally, the **pulse rate** is the same as the heart rate. The normal pulse has a fairly regular rhythm with evenly spaced beats. It varies slightly with breathing.

Blood pressure

A considerable head of pressure is required to keep blood flowing at an adequate rate through the miles of blood vessels offering resistance to flow. A severed artery will squirt blood several feet into the air! Traditionally, blood pressure is expressed in terms of how high a column of mercury it can, theoretically, support (mercury is 13 times heavier than blood).

Arterial blood pressure is not constant. When the left ventricle contracts and ejects blood (a phase in the heart's pumping cycle called **systole**), the pressure in the large arteries rises to a peak, the **systolic pressure,** typically 120 millimetres (mm) of mercury (usually written 120mmHg). When the ventricle relaxes and the heart receives the inflowing venous blood (a phase called **diastole**), the arterial blood pressure falls, but not to zero. The 'elastic bag' effect of the larger arteries ensures that adequate pressure is maintained to keep the blood circulating after the aortic valve has closed. The lowest pressure (**diastolic**) in the main arteries is typically 80mmHg.

Thus, a typical blood pressure might be expressed in the form 120/80 (i.e. systolic/diastolic).

Water flow in the tissues

Just as the pressure in a plumbing system drops progressively throughout its length, so the passage of blood through the branches of the arterial tree is accompanied by a drop in blood pressure. The blood pressures at the arterial and venous ends of a tissue capillary are typically 32mmHg and 12mmHg respectively. This so-called **hydrostatic pressure** tends to push fluid out into the interstitial fluid space. But it is opposed by another force.

In the tissues, water and most of the substances dissolved in it pass freely between plasma and interstitial fluid. However, plasma has a very slightly higher osmotic pressure that tends to draw water out of the interstitial space. This small unique additional force, called the **plasma oncotic pressure**, is due mainly to plasma proteins, particularly albumin. The protein molecules are mostly too large to pass through the normal capillary wall and therefore cause additional osmotic pressure within the vascular system. The plasma oncotic pressure is normally 25mmHg. Fluid flows out of the capillary at the arterial end where the hydrostatic pressure is higher and flows back at the venous end where the oncotic pressure dominates; the net result is a circulation of fluid in the interstitial spaces surrounding the cells.

Excess interstitial fluid drains into **lymphatic vessels**, capillary-like channels starting in the tissue spaces and forming their own separate network. They also carry debris and organisms arising from local damage, infection or inflammation. The lymphatic vessels connect to a series of **lymph nodes**, commonly referred to as glands (superficial ones can sometimes be felt as small hard round lumps under the skin, particularly in the neck and groin). The nodes filter and process debris and pass the fluid (**lymph**) on to progressively more structured lymphatic vessels which eventually drain into large veins deep in the lower neck.

Disorders causing an increase in capillary hydrostatic pressure, a decrease in plasma albumin or a blockage in lymphatic drainage encourage water to accumulate in the interstitial space. In these circumstances the tissues become swollen and boggy in texture, a condition known as **oedema**.

The above account does not apply to the lungs. The blood pressure in the pulmonary circulation is much lower than that in the systemic circulation, and the hydrostatic pressure in the lung capillaries is lower than the plasma oncotic pressure.

Heart failure

Let us now consider what happens when the heart fails to pump sufficient blood to meet the needs of the body, a condition called heart failure (**cardiac failure**). The term usually refers to a partial failure of the pump; complete failure is rapidly fatal. The effects depend on the nature, location, extent and rate of onset of the causative lesion (damage), but some general points can be made to illustrate concepts introduced above.

In **left ventricular failure** (left heart failure) the cardiac output falls causing a reduction in tissue blood flow (**perfusion**). Perfusion of skin and muscle is reduced giving rise to cold skin and fatigue. If the cardiac output is severely reduced, the functioning of vital organs such as the brain and kidney may be seriously affected. The failing left heart also impedes the return of blood from the lungs, causing a rise in the blood pressure of the pulmonary (lung) vessels, which become congested. In sudden (**acute**) left ventricular failure, the lung capillary hydrostatic pressure may exceed the opposing plasma oncotic pressure sufficiently to cause oedema of the lungs (**pulmonary oedema**). This impairs gas exchange and causes breathlessness.

Heart failure is often more generalised and the flow of blood from the great veins into the right heart may also be impeded causing venous congestion in the systemic circulation. The hydrostatic pressure in the tissue capillaries may rise sufficiently to cause oedema, particularly in the lowest regions of the body, seen typically as swollen ankles and legs. This is **congestive cardiac failure**. There are other causes of oedema apart from heart failure, and swollen feet and ankles can occur in normal people who stand for long periods.

Other mechanisms also contribute to water and salt retention in heart failure, and an appreciation of these is important in selecting the right treatment.

———— Organs and systems ————

An **organ** is a discrete (that is, separate and distinct) structural unit performing particular functions for the body. It may contain a number of different tissues or cells, but usually one specialised form predominates. We have already studied one organ, the heart; other examples are the lungs, liver, kidneys, stomach, pancreas, bowels, brain, uterus, gonads, etc. An organ is part of a **system**, a higher level of organisation involving other structures, even other organs. For instance, the heart and the system of blood vessels is referred to as the **cardiovascular system**, the whole system being required to circulate blood around the body. Some organs are involved in the operations of more than one system.

The lungs and the respiratory system

Respiration is the uptake of oxygen and expulsion of carbon dioxide.

Cells take up oxygen, use it to release energy from food fuels and, in the process, produce carbon dioxide. The dissolved gases are exchanged between cytoplasm and interstitial fluid. This is respiration at cellular level. The term respiration is also applied to the exchange of oxygen and carbon dioxide between blood and air.

The **respiratory system** comprises the lungs and the air passages connecting them to the outside. It brings fresh air into close proximity with the blood capillaries of the lungs and provides an efficient means of gas exchange.

The lungs and diaphragm were briefly mentioned earlier (see figure 2.3, page 11). The upper air passages leading from the mouth and nose warm and moisten the air on its way to the lungs. In the neck, air is conducted through the **larynx** to the windpipe (**trachea**). The larynx is the hard gristly structure that can be felt at the front of the neck, most prominently as the Adam's apple. It contains the vocal cords. The top of the trachea lies beneath the larynx just behind the notch at the top of the breast bone. From here the trachea passes downwards 10 centimetres (cm) into the thoracic cavity where it divides into two short tubes, the left and right main **bronchi** (singular, bronchus), supplying the left and right lungs respectively (see figure 2.10). The bronchi branch many times, rather like trees, until the air passages end in thousands of minute tubes called **bronchioles** which carry air to and from the structures in which gas exchange actually occurs, the **acini.**

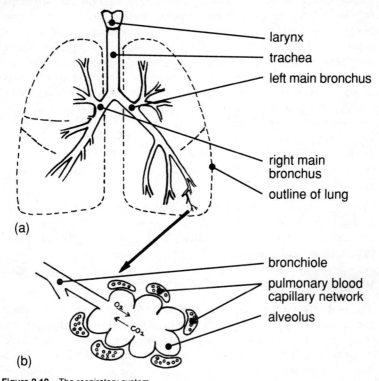

(a)

(b)

larynx
trachea
left main bronchus
right main bronchus
outline of lung

bronchiole
pulmonary blood capillary network
alveolus

Figure 2.10 The respiratory system
(**a**) Main air passages and outline of the lungs.
(**b**) Magnified view of gas exchange unit (acinus).

As shown in figure 2.10, the **acinus** contains air chambers, the smallest units of which are the **alveoli**. These are lined with a very thin epithelium through which gases pass rapidly to and from a dense network of closely applied pulmonary capillaries. A pair of adult lungs contains hundreds of millions of alveoli; the total surface available for gas exchange is equivalent to half the area of a tennis court.

When the alveoli expand, air is drawn into the lungs (**inhalation** or **inspiration**); when they shrink, due to contraction of the elastic fibres in their walls, air is expelled (**exhalation** or **expiration**).

At this microscopic level, the thin liquid film on the surfaces exerts a relatively powerful force called surface tension. Unopposed, it could cause the alveoli to remain permanently collapsed. This is prevented by a substance called **pulmonary surfactant** which lines the epithelium, reduces surface tension and allows the lung to expand again on inspiration. It is made by special cells scattered among the respiratory epithelium. Production starts just before birth. In a few babies the process is still immature at birth. They may temporarily make insufficient surfactant and may develop the **respiratory distress syndrome**, a condition in which the lungs tend to remain collapsed and airless. Treatment with an artificial surfactant is available.

The oxygen and carbon dioxide levels in arterial blood are normally kept within certain limits. This is achieved by appropriate adjustment of the rate and volume of air flow (**ventilation**) in the lungs.

Ventilation

The volume of the air passages in which gas-exchange does not occur is called the **dead space**, typically 150ml. In order to get sufficient fresh air into the acini to meet the needs of respiration, larger amounts must be breathed. The volume normally inhaled in each breath is called the **tidal volume**, usually about 450ml in an adult at rest. The amount of air exchanged over a period of time also depends on how frequently we breathe (**respiratory rate**), typically about 16 breaths per minute. An important practical measurement is the **minute volume**, the amount inhaled, or exhaled, in a minute; it is equal to the respiratory rate multiplied by the tidal volume.

Normal quiet breathing involves contraction and relaxation of the muscles of the diaphragm. Deeper breathing is assisted by muscles attached to the chest wall. The additional air needed to supply more oxygen to the body during physical exertion is obtained by increasing the tidal volume and the respiratory rate.

After exhalation there is still a large amount of gas left in the lungs. Its composition is not the same as air because of the gas-exchange that has already occurred. Fresh incoming air mixes with residual gas in the acini to form an intermediary mixture.

Gas pressure

The pressures (**tensions**) of a gas on either side of the alveolar wall affect the net direction of flow. Molecules in a gas are in a constant state of motion. The more present, the greater the number of impacts against adjacent surfaces, the greater the pressure exerted on those surfaces and, in the case of a gas permeable barrier, the larger the number likely to shoot through the pores to the other side (**diffusion**). The principle applies whether the molecules are free in a volume of gas or dissolved in a volume of fluid.

The total pressure exerted by a mixture of gases, such as air, is the sum of all the individual gas pressures (**partial pressures**). The atmospheric, or barometric, pressure of air at sea level varies slightly but is usually around 760mmHg. Oxygen accounts for one-fifth of the volume of fresh warm moist air entering the lungs and, therefore, for one-fifth of the total gas pressure. Thus, after inhalation the partial pressure of oxygen entering the lower air passages is normally 150mmHg.

After mixing with residual lung gases the average partial pressure of oxygen in the alveolus is about 100mmHg. The oxygen pressure (tension) in the de-oxygenated blood returning from the tissues to the lungs (via the heart) is about 40mmHg. The net effect is that oxygen passes from the alveolar air into the pulmonary capillary blood. Gas exchange is so efficient that the oxygen tension in the blood leaving the lungs and passing through the heart into the systemic arteries is normally about 95mmHg.

It is gas pressure that forces oxygen from plasma into the tissues. But oxygen is not very soluble and plasma can only hold a limited amount at any instant. Most of the oxygen in blood is held by haemoglobin acting as a vast reservoir which feeds the gas to the plasma.

Carbon dioxide pressure in the blood returning to the lungs is higher than that in the air-freshened alveoli. The gas flows into the lungs and is expelled from the body by exhalation.

The gas levels in arterial blood also provide automatic feed-back control of respiration. A rise in carbon dioxide tension or a fall in oxygen tension stimulate ventilation.

A state called **respiratory failure** is said to be present when, due to lung disease, the oxygen tension in arterial blood falls below 60mmHg. It is potentially dangerous. Coma occurs at 30mmHg.

The alimentary system (digestive tract)

The alimentary system is essentially a long tube running through the body. It receives food at one end, extracts nutrients and expels the unwanted residue in faeces at the other end. Parts of the tube have taken on specialised forms and functions. The anatomical arrangement is outlined in figure 2.11. The epithelial cells lining the inside of the tract are derived from the embryonic endoderm. In the stomach and intestines they become highly specialised. Early in development parts of the tract sprout sideways to form the liver and pancreas; they remain connected to the small bowel by their ducts.

The teeth and tongue, aided by saliva, pulp food into a soft round mass (**bolus**). The act of swallowing propels the bolus down the gullet (**oesophagus**) into the stomach, which lies just under the diaphragm. Complex foods are progressively broken down (**digested**) in the stomach and small bowel (**small intestine**) by digestive juices containing specific enzymes.

Special epithelial cells in the stomach produce hydrochloric acid (H-Cl) and an enzyme called pepsin which partially degrade food protein. Other cells make a layer of mucus containing an antacid (bicarbonate) to protect the lining of the stomach from also being digested.

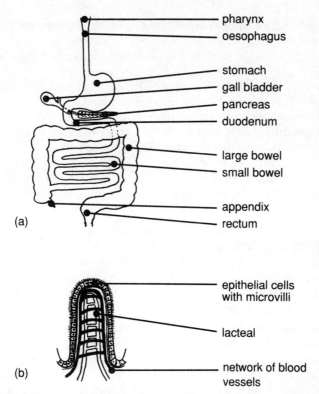

pharynx
oesophagus

stomach
gall bladder
pancreas
duodenum

large bowel
small bowel

appendix
rectum

(a)

epithelial cells
with microvilli

lacteal

network of blood
vessels

(b)

Figure 2.11 The alimentary canal
(a) The organs
(b) Structure of a small bowel villus.

Some digestive juices are formed outside the main tract and flow through ducts into the initial part of the small bowel (the **duodenum**) just beyond the stomach. These are the bile and the pancreatic juices. Bile is formed in the liver and stored in the gall bladder ready to be released after a meal. It contains the **bile acids** which emulsify fats into tiny, more digestible, particles. Pancreatic juice is formed in the pancreas, an organ lying close to the duodenum. It produces enzymes to digest proteins, fats and complex sugars, and bicarbonate to neutralise acid from the stomach. The small bowel also makes its own digestive juice which contains yet more enzymes to further break down the partially digested food materials.

Suitable products of digestion are absorbed in the small intestine. The small bowel is about five metres long and its internal surface is covered with tiny finger-like projections (**villi**) which greatly increase the area for absorption (see figure 2.11). The villi are covered with special epithelial cells which, in turn, have microvilli on their free surfaces to further increase the absorptive area. The cells selectively pass the nutrients from the lumen of the intestine to vessels inside the villi. For instance, simple sugars and amino acids pass into blood capillaries which drain into the **portal system**, a special venous system carrying blood directly to the liver. The epithelial cells absorb degraded fats and reassemble them into larger fat particles which then pass into the **lacteals**, lymphatic vessels in the villi, which eventually drain into the ordinary venous system like other lymphatics.

Unabsorbed food and fluid eventually passes into the large bowel (**large intestine**, or **colon**) which absorbs water and salts and processes the waste matter into semi-solid faeces. At the end of the colon is the rectum which contains the last cavity of the alimentary canal. The rectum expels faeces from the body through the anus.

The **appendix** is a small worm-like tubular structure communicating with the large bowel near its junction with the small bowel; the free end is blind (see figure 2.11 page 37). Its importance lies in its tendency to obstruction and infection, which can lead to **acute appendicitis**, the commonest abdominal surgical emergency in the UK.

Normally, food passes through the alimentary canal in one direction. This is achieved by the rhythmical propulsive action (**peristalsis**) of muscles in the canal wall, and by the presence of special muscular valves (**sphincters**) at the entrances to the stomach, duodenum and colon. Food is retained for various lengths of time in different parts of the tract to ensure complete processing. The stomach may take many hours to release its contents after a large meal.

The liver

The liver is the body's major chemical factory. Its many functions can be largely categorised under the headings: chemical processing (including detoxification), storage, manufacture and supply. It receives oxygenated arterial blood from the

hepatic artery and venous blood directly from the stomach and intestines via the **portal vein**. Blood leaves the liver through the **hepatic vein** which drains into the inferior vena cava. Most of the chemical activities occur in the **parenchymal cells** (or **hepatocytes**) which are the most abundant cells in the liver.

The internal architecture of the organ is complicated but it can be represented functionally as a vast number of small blood passages passing through sheets of parenchymal cells, thus providing a large area for the exchange of materials (a familiar concept). The blood passages are called **sinusoids**; they are larger than capillaries. Blood from the portal venous system passes along the sinusoid and drains into a tributary of the hepatic vein.

A separate system of ducts carrying bile originates from the parenchymal tissue.

The portal venous system carries absorbed toxins (toxic substances), drugs, alcohol and food products, such as amino acids and sugars, from the digestive tract to the liver for processing. The liver can often modify toxic molecules to make them less harmful and/or make them more amenable to removal by the kidneys.

The liver is involved in the metabolism of amino acids. Depending on the body's needs, it may use them to make proteins, pass them into the general circulation for utilisation by other tissues, or convert them to glucose when fuel supplies are low. It also converts unwanted amino acid nitrogen into **urea**, as mentioned earlier on page 9 (also see figure 2.1 page 7).

The liver provides a continuous supply of glucose to the rest of the body. After a meal some of the absorbed glucose passes into the general circulation and some is stored in the liver in the form of **glycogen**, a large molecular complex consisting of many glucose units joined together chemically (it is the animal equivalent of starch). In between meals, when the blood glucose levels fall, the liver breaks down glycogen and releases glucose as required into the circulation. Glycogen stores last for less than a day. Once they are depleted, as may occur after fasting or in starvation, the body starts to break down its own protein into amino acids, which can be converted into glucose.

Red blood cells live for about 110 days after which they are destroyed. One of the break-down products of haemoglobin is **bilirubin**, a yellow pigment found in bile. The parenchymal cells of the liver extract bilirubin from plasma, in which it is carried by albumin, and convert it into a more water soluble form which passes into the bile ducts and eventually into the duodenum. In certain diseases bilirubin accumulates in the blood and tissues and causes **jaundice**, a yellow discoloration of the skin.

Other functions of the liver include storage of iron and vitamins (especially A, D and B_{12}), metabolism of **lipids** (fats and related substances) and the manufacture of bile acids and plasma proteins (including albumin and blood clotting factors, but not antibodies).

Like most major organs, the liver has plenty of spare capacity to deal with excessive demands. It is also capable of regenerating itself after injury. But extensive disease and damage can lead to **hepatic failure**, a life-threatening condition.

The kidneys

The kidneys are bean-shaped organs at the back of the abdominal cavity (see figure 2.3, page 11). They remove unwanted substances from the blood and discharge them from the body as urine. Figure 2.12 shows the plumbing arrangement in the male.

The kidneys account for only 0.5 per cent of body weight but they receive, via the **renal arteries**, at least a fifth of the heart's total output of blood. They filter much of this blood through a sieve which allows most substances to pass, except blood cells and plasma proteins. The filtered fluid (**filtrate**) is effectively plasma without its proteins. The kidneys filter a fifth of the incoming plasma, typically producing 120ml of filtrate per minute (this is an important measurement known as the **glomerular filtration rate**, or **gfr**). They then extract from the filtrate all the substances that need to be conserved and pass them back into the blood stream. Thus, the filtrate

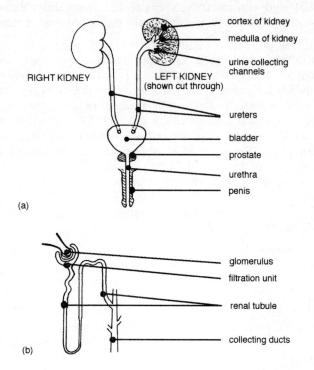

Figure 2.12 The kidneys and urinary tract
(a) Male urinary tract
(b) Microscopic structure of a nephron

turns into urine, which contains the remaining unwanted substances, such as urea. Each day the kidneys filter about 180 litres of plasma and form approximately one to two litres of urine, so about 99 per cent of the filtered water is taken back into the body, fortunately.

Cleansed blood passes back into the general circulation via the renal veins. The urine from each kidney flows continuously down a tube (**ureter**) to the **bladder**, which is a muscular-walled reservoir. At intervals, and under conscious control, the bladder discharges urine to the outside through a single tube known as the **urethra**. In men the urethra passes through the **prostate** (a gland contributing to the liquid component of semen) and then the penis (see figure 2.12). In women it does not pass through such structures and is much shorter at four centimetres. The passage from the kidney to the end of the urethra is often referred to as the **urinary tract**.

The microscopic units responsible for filtering blood and forming urine are the **nephrons**; there are a million in each kidney. They each comprise a filtration unit and a **tubule**, a narrow tube with walls consisting of a single layer of specialised epithelial cells (see figure 2.12 page 41). The tubule begins with a blind end in the outer region (**cortex**) of the kidney. The filtration unit consists of a knot of capillaries (a **glomerulus**) enveloped in an expanded bag of epithelium at the blind end of the tubule. The hydrostatic pressure in the glomerular capillaries is relatively high and it forces the blood filtrate into the lumen of the tubule. The biochemistry and physiology of the renal tubule is complicated. A simplified account follows.

Bulk exchanges of material between the filtrate and the epithelial cells, and between the epithelial cells and another capillary network, occur in the first part of the renal tubule. Thus, all the glucose and amino acids, 90 per cent of the salts and 85 per cent of the water in the filtrate pass back into the blood stream. Some materials pass the other way (from blood to filtrate), for instance some drug derivatives formed in the liver.

The last part of the tubule (and its immediate connecting duct in the core of the kidney) fine tunes the composition of the urine according to needs. Under the influence of **antidiuretic hormone** (**ADH**), it regulates the amount of water in the plasma and interstitial fluid. ADH comes from the pea-sized **pituitary gland** attached to the underside of the brain. When we are thirsty and in need of water the pituitary releases ADH into the blood stream. The kidneys respond by reabsorbing more water from the filtrate. The opposite happens when we drink more than we need. Thus, when we are water-deprived we make small amounts of concentrated urine, and when we drink too much water we excrete it in large volumes of dilute urine. An increased flow of urine is called a **diuresis**.

In terms of total dissolved substances, the kidney can form urine with concentrations ranging from a quarter to four times that of the filtered plasma. Urea is excreted with great efficiency, its concentration in urine can be up to a hundred times that in plasma. As we have seen, other substances are conserved and do not appear in urine.

Under the influence of other hormones (e.g. **aldosterone** see chapter nine, page 210), the renal tubule also controls the excretion of sodium and potassium and their concentrations in plasma. Sodium is very important in the maintenance of osmotic pressure in the tissues and it greatly influences the distribution of water. The kidneys ensure that a favourable and constant sodium concentration is maintained in plasma, and therefore in interstitial fluid, to provide the environment necessary for normal cell function. The concentration of potassium in plasma is much lower than that of sodium. It is tightly regulated; abnormally high or low levels can be dangerous. The kidneys also help to control the acidity of the blood (see page 48).

Under normal circumstances the kidneys easily cope with the needs of the body – in fact, one healthy kidney can. Some diseases damage the kidneys and affect their ability to function properly. When renal function deteriorates to such an extent that unwanted substances accumulate excessively in the blood (**uraemia**) the patient is said to be in a state of **renal failure**. Untreated, severe renal failure is life-threatening. **Dialysis** is an artificial method used to remove unwanted waste substances from the blood when the kidneys fail. Some patients with permanent renal failure have been successfully treated for years using dialysis techniques. However, dialysis does not perform all the functions of the normal kidney and additional treatments are required to combat other complications of renal disease.

The brain

In the most primitive animals it is the outer layer that provides contact with, and appreciation of, the outside world. This is reflected in our embryonic development which, in the early stages, appears to mimic our evolution from simpler life forms. The ectoderm gives rise to the skin and the nervous system. A strip of ectoderm running lengthways infolds forming a separate tube under the remaining ectoderm, which closes up again (see figure 2.6, page 19). This **neural tube** develops into the central controlling and co-ordinating part of the nervous system (**central nervous system** or **CNS**). At one end the tube undergoes extensive changes to become the brain, the remainder becomes the spinal cord.

Appreciation of the outside world comes largely from structures at or near the surface of the body, such as the skin (touch) and the special sense organs like the nose, ear and eye. These send nerve impulses, essentially digital electrical signals, to the CNS for interpretation. There are also nerve connections from the CNS to motor structures, such as muscles, so that appropriate responses can be made.

The brain is also the seat of memory, thought, consciousness and emotion.

Neurons: white and grey matter

The neuron (nerve cell) was introduced earlier. Numerous projections extend from the cell body (see figure 2.7, page 20). One of them is the **axon**, which transmits signals *away* from the main body of the neuron *to* other neurons, or to cells that perform specific actions on receiving the signal (e.g. muscle cells). Axons are the basic nerve fibres. They can be very long and are bundled into tracts, forming the so-called **white matter** of the CNS (brain and spinal cord), and into the nerves of the **peripheral nervous system** (the nervous system outside the CNS). The other projections are called **dendrites**. They receive signals *from* other neurons or specialised receptor (sense) cells and transmit them *towards* the main body of the neuron.

In the brain, neuron cell bodies are clustered together to form regions of **grey matter**, the largest and most complex of which is the **cerebral cortex**. There are (approximately!) 50 thousand million neurons in the human brain and a single neuron may have over 5,000 connections with other neurons. The networks of interconnections are incredibly complex and highly organised, and there are many specialised regions within the brain subserving particular functions.

Anatomy of the cerebral hemispheres

The brain occupies most of the upper half of the head and is protected by a bony case, the **cranium**. The upper part of the brain is split into separate left and right halves, the **cerebral hemispheres**, which look rather like two very large dumplings pushed close together. The outermost layer of the hemispheres consists of the grey matter of the cerebral cortex. Only a third of the cortex can be seen on the surface because it is folded into a series of outward bulges (**convolutions**) and deep grooves (**fissures** or **sulci**).

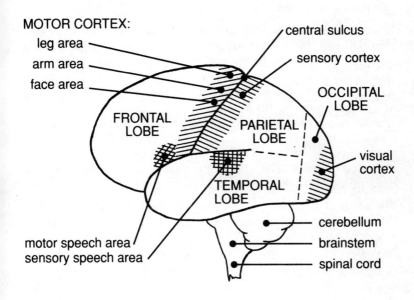

Figure 2.13 The brain – left side

Figure 2.13 shows some of the features of the human cerebral cortex (for clarity, the convolutions are omitted). Each cerebral hemisphere is divided into four major anatomical regions, the **frontal**, **parietal**, **occipital** and **temporal lobes**, which lie under cranial bones of the same name. Note that the **central sulcus** demarcates the frontal lobe, which lies in front of it, and the parietal lobe, which lies behind it.

The motor and sensory cortex

The strip of frontal lobe immediately anterior to (in front of) the central sulcus contains the **motor area** which drives the muscles of the opposite side of the body. The part responsible for movement of the lower limb is represented at the top and that responsible for upper limb movement is situated further down (see figure 2.13); in fact, the body segments are represented upside-down.

Many of the nerve tracts carrying signals to and from the cortex cross over to the opposite side at some point in the central nervous system. The long axons of the cortical motor neurons pass through the interior of the hemisphere and continue downwards into the **brain stem**, an important section of the brain that connects the two cerebral hemispheres above with the spinal cord below. At the lower end of the brain stem these motor fibres cross over to the opposite side before continuing their journey downwards to relay with **lower motor neurons** in the spinal cord. The axons of the lower motor neurons communicate with muscle fibres via the peripheral nerves.

The strip of parietal lobe behind the central sulcus contains the **sensory area** which is concerned with the interpretation of incoming sensation, such as recognising which part of the body has been touched. Like the motor cortex, it serves the opposite side of the body, which is represented upside-down.

The special senses of the head are subserved in other regions of the cerebral cortex. That responsible for vision is in the posterior part of the occipital lobe.

The dominant hemisphere and the speech centres

The specialised areas of cortex described above are present in both hemispheres, but the centres responsible for language are found only in one, the so-called **dominant hemisphere**.

This is the left cerebral hemisphere in right-handed people, and the right in some, but not all, left-handers.

Language input is processed and interpreted in specialised areas of the dominant hemisphere, such as the sensory speech centre (**Wernicke's area**). In front of the motor cortex there is a motor speech centre (**Broca's area**) responsible for language output; its signals pass to the motor cortex for expression as speech.

——— Integration of the whole ———

Mind and body are closely linked. Problems with one invariably affect the other. The nervous system pervades almost all tissues and organs. The **autonomic nervous system** provides automatic control of bodily functions (e.g. breathing, heart beat, gastro-intestinal function, etc.). Most of the time we are unaware of its activities. We shall revisit the brain-body connection in chapter five.

Maintenance of physical health requires the integrated action of the life support systems. We have seen how the kidneys, hormone-producing glands and the blood circulation work together to control water and salt levels in the body. The remaining sections of this chapter elaborate on this theme and introduce additional topics of importance in medicine.

Acidity and hydrogen ions

In pure water approximately two out of every thousand million H_2O molecules split (**dissociate**) into positively charged hydrogen ions (H^+) and negatively charged hydroxyl ions (OH^-; the oxygen atom is still chemically bonded to one hydrogen atom but its second bond is now free and forms a negative charge). Acidity is due to an excess of hydrogen ions in solution. Alkalinity is due to an excess of hydroxyl ions. Pure water is neutral, neither acid nor alkaline, because it contains equal numbers of hydrogen and hydroxyl ions; and it is bland because it forms so few. When acids like hydrogen chloride (H-Cl) dissolve in water they dissociate, flooding the solution with hydrogen ions. The corrosive nature of such strong acids is due to the vast number of hydrogen ions made available to react chemically with other substances. As the hydrogen-ion concentration increases, fewer water molecules dissociate and the hydroxyl-ion concentration falls. The opposite happens in alkaline solutions, which therefore contain lower hydrogen-ion concentrations than pure water. Plasma and the interstitial fluid bathing the cells are very slightly alkaline. Hydrogen-ion concentration is often expressed as a pH value, which is a negative logarithmic function of concentration. The pH scale ranges from 0 to 14 where 0 represents extreme acidity and 14 represents extreme alkalinity. The pH of pure water is 7 (neutral), and the pH of blood is normally 7.4.

To function normally, and live, the cells require a particular and very stable hydrogen-ion environment. Metabolism continuously produces large amounts of hydrogen ion which, unchecked, could cause a dangerous increase in acidity. The combined efforts of the lungs, kidneys and circulation ensure that the plasma hydrogen-ion concentration is tightly controlled.

Carbon dioxide is a major product of the metabolism of sugars, fats and amino acids. It reacts with water to form **carbonic acid** (H_2CO_3), which is a weak acid because it dissociates only to a limited extent, forming hydrogen ions and bicarbonate ions. Like the hydroxyl ion, bicarbonate (HCO_3^-) is a group of atoms with a negative charge. These events (**reactions**) can be summarised chemically as follows:

$$CO_2 + H_2O \rightleftharpoons H_2CO_3 \rightleftharpoons H^+ + HCO_3^-$$

carbon + water $\rightleftharpoons$ carbonic $\rightleftharpoons$ hydrogen + bicarbonate
dioxide   acid   ion

The symbol $\rightleftharpoons$ indicates that the reaction may go from left to right, or right to left, depending on prevailing conditions.

It is through this series of reactions that the blood, lungs and kidneys effectively control the hydrogen-ion concentration. When blood reaches the lungs, carbon dioxide gas is removed by ventilation, thereby pulling the reaction to the left. The kidney tubules can excrete hydrogen ions into the urine, and they make bicarbonate, which is reabsorbed back into the blood stream. Between them, the kidneys and lungs maintain fairly constant levels of bicarbonate and carbonic acid in plasma, in a molecular ratio of about twenty to one. The bicarbonate can react immediately with excess hydrogen ions, effectively neutralising (buffering) them until they reach the lungs and kidneys for disposal.

An increase in the concentration of carbon dioxide or hydrogen ion in plasma stimulates special areas of the brain responsible for the control of respiration (**respiratory centres**). Nerves from these centres pass motor signals to the diaphragm, which in turn increases ventilation. This provides a sensitive rapid-response mechanism for the control of hydrogen ions.

There is another twist to the story. In the tissues, carbon dioxide passes into the red blood cells where it forms hydrogen ions (the same reactions as those seen above). Haemoglobin takes up the hydrogen ions, effectively neutralising (buffering) them, but as a consequence its ability to hold oxygen decreases. Oxygen then flows out of the capillaries to the tissues. In the lungs these events are reversed.

The control of plasma glucose

A continuous supply of glucose to the brain is essential. Without it, coma occurs within minutes.

Two hormones from the pancreas regulate the uptake, storage and release of glucose in the liver, thereby controlling its concentration in the blood stream (see figure 2.14). They are the proteins **insulin** and **glucagon** (not to be confused with glycogen, the polymer of glucose stored in the liver). These chemical messengers arise from special groups of cells quite separate from those producing the pancreatic digestive enzymes and they pass directly into the blood stream. A low plasma glucose concentration stimulates the **A** cells of the pancreas to release glucagon which, on reaching the liver, accelerates the rate of glucose production from glycogen. A high plasma glucose stimulates the pancreatic **B** cells to produce insulin which in turn stimulates the liver to convert glucose into glycogen. Insulin also increases glucose uptake into muscle and fat cells. These mechanisms combine to form a feed-back control system which maintains healthy plasma glucose levels. Adrenaline and some other hormones also affect plasma glucose levels.

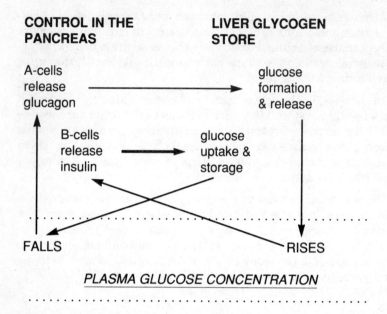

Figure 2.14 Hormonal control of plasma glucose

Insulin deficiency causes **diabetes mellitus**, a condition characterised by abnormally high plasma glucose levels (see page 100).

Homeostasis

The maintenance of a healthy steady state of metabolism and the tendency to correct potentially harmful changes is known as **homeostasis**.

Hundreds of feed-back control systems regulate the body's chemical and physiological activities. Like all good control systems, they work economically. A few nerve impulses or a few hormone molecules can induce big changes in receptive target tissues and organs. Each hormone acts selectively, inducing particular effects, in particular cells. This **specificity** is due to the presence in the cell of unique molecular receptors (proteins) which recognise and respond to particular hormones, the 'lock and key' principle again.

Humans generally reach peak physical performance in their second and third decades. As age advances further there is a gradual decline in the efficiency of some organs, but usually the normal needs of the body can still be met easily. Homeostatic control mechanisms continue to maintain vital internal environmental conditions (e.g. plasma gas, salt and hydrogen-ion levels) within tight limits into (healthy) old age.

Homeostasis operates at all levels of organisation, from molecular to behavioural.

3
DISEASE

Introduction

What is disease?

There is no entirely satisfactory definition. Disease might be defined as an abnormality of bodily form or function that causes an adverse or unfavourable effect. The distinction of disease from health, and the abnormal from the normal, is not always easy. In any large group of apparently healthy people there will be variations in the form and functioning of tissues and organs, and in the response to physical and mental stress and injury. A gradual deterioration of tissue and organ function appears to be part of the normal aging process. Some people are much less fit than others but they are not necessarily sick or incapacitated, although in certain circumstances they might be disadvantaged.

The terms disease, disorder and condition are often used interchangeably in medical texts, and they are to some extent in this book. The word **condition**, rather than **disease**, is usually applied to biological variations that have no obvious adverse effect. The term **syndrome** is commonly used in medicine. It refers to a set of symptoms or signs that occur in combination and suggest a particular disease, disorder or condition. In practice the word disease is more often applied to conditions in which the disease process is still active. Thus, deformity and disability caused by an injury during birth might not be regarded as a disease.

Nearly half of this chapter is devoted to atherosclerosis and cancer, disease processes responsible for two-thirds of all deaths in the UK and US.

Measuring disease

The study of the occurrence and distribution of diseases in populations (**epidemiology**) can yield valuable information. It may suggest possible causes, indicate important changes and provide data required for decision-making in areas such as public health and government expenditure. Reliable data are required to produce meaningful statistics. Valid comparisons of data collected at different times, in different studies, in different populations and by different investigators require a consistent use of definitions for diseases and disease parameters. National statistics on causes of death are based on the information provided by doctors on death certificates. Death certificate entries (should) follow certain guidelines so that diseases can be accurately categorized. Traditions in diagnostic labelling sometimes differ, especially between countries, making some comparisons difficult. Clinicians occasionally make mistakes in diagnosis and enter erroneous data, but national data bases are usually so large that the effects are diluted to insignificance.

Mortality statistics are concerned with the rates, risks and causes of death. Morbidity statistics such as prevalence and incidence are measures of the occurrence of diseases in communities. These terms have precise meanings in epidemiology. A clear understanding of the definitions is required to make valid deductions and predictions from the data. This book aims to convey the gist of relevant statistics without detailed definition of technical terms.

Cause, effect and association

In many diseases, such as **coronary atherosclerosis**, there is a chain of causes and effects, one thing leading to another, between the very first pathological change and the final full-blown clinical event. The initiating cause of a disease may not be known, even though much may be known about the subsequent changes and the pathological processes involved. Theories regarding causes are usually rigorously tested before they are accepted as fact. Discovery of cause provides a rational basis for the development of preventive measures and curative treatments.

Sometimes epidemiological or clinical studies on groups of people or patients with particular characteristics, in particular areas, on particular foods etc., show an association between the occurrence of one or more factors and the occurrence of a disease. This is a statistical association and it does not necessarily mean that a particular factor is the cause of the disease, but it may provide an important clue. For instance, a study on disease X, dietary fat intake and fatness in a large population might show a strong statistical association between the disease and both of the factors. This does not mean that obesity causes the disease. Overeating fat might cause both obesity and disease X. Alternatively, the cause might be an unknown factor which tends to alter in relation to dietary fat intake. Initiation or progression of the disease may require the interaction of several factors, of which diet may be just one. Sometimes the association of a particular factor with the development of a disease is so overwhelming that there is little doubt that it is the main cause – for example, smoking and lung cancer in the UK. Factors that increase the chances of contracting a disease are known as **risk factors**.

Classification of disease

Diseases can be listed or classified by cause, disease process, system and organ, clinical symptoms and syndromes, frequency of occurrence, seriousness, economic importance, or in a form useful for diagnosis. In practice disease classification utilises several of these elements. No single system is entirely satisfactory for all purposes. A common method considers each body system and organ in turn and then subdivides the diseases affecting them into groups by cause or disease process. This provides a reasonably complete listing but gaps in knowledge can lead to inconsistencies and there is a degree of overlap and duplication; some diseases affect more than one system and some have more than one cause.

The term **idiopathic** refers to a disorder with unknown cause. **Iatrogenic** refers to disease caused by the doctor. In medicine the words **acute** and **chronic** are used to categorise diseases by their time courses, referring to illnesses of short and long duration respectively.

—— Diseases of the blood vessels ——

Introduction

In this section we shall concentrate mainly, but not exclusively, on **atherosclerosis**, a particularly important disease process affecting the arterial wall. It is the medical scourge of western civilisation, the pathology behind most cases of heart disease and stroke.

Atherosclerosis (or **atheroma**) is a thickening of the arterial wall due to deposits, (**plaques**), consisting of **lipid** (fats, cholesterol) and other complex materials in the layers beneath the endothelium (see figure 3.1). As the disease progresses the blood channel (lumen) may become seriously narrowed by the obtruding lesions. The precise cause and mechanism of plaque formation are still not completely understood.

Certain events that can occur on the atherosclerotic plaque are of considerable clinical importance (see figure 3.1). Damaged endothelium and exposed plaque material attract platelets which adhere to the vessel wall and initiate the formation of a fibrin clot. The process may continue until a blood clot (**thrombus**) is formed, which may be limited and eventually resolve and become part of the plaque, or may extend further into the lumen and obstruct blood flow.

Atherosclerosis has a predilection for particular parts of the arterial tree, such as the aorta and the arteries supplying the heart, brain and legs. Even within these vessels the lesions occur mostly at favoured sites, such as branch points and sharp bends.

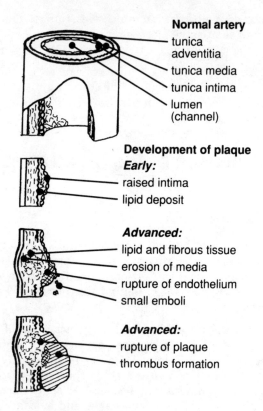

Normal artery

tunica adventitia

tunica media

tunica intima

lumen (channel)

Development of plaque

Early:

raised intima

lipid deposit

Advanced:

lipid and fibrous tissue

erosion of media

rupture of endothelium

small emboli

Advanced:

rupture of plaque

thrombus formation

Figure 3.1 Development of atherosclerosis

Ischaemia is an inadequate supply of blood (and oxygen) to a part, due to narrowing or obstruction of the arterial lumen, such as occurs in atherosclerosis. It may lead to varying degrees of dysfunction or disability in the part of the body affected, and is often accompanied by pain. Severe ischaemia can cause cell death (**necrosis**), resulting in a localised region of dead tissue known as an **infarct** (the process is called **infarction**). Heart attacks are often due to **myocardial infarction** (infarction of the heart muscle).

Thrombosis refers to the formation or presence of a blood clot in the circulatory system. It may be arterial, as in **coronary thrombosis** (of the coronary arteries, leading to myocardial infarction), or venous, as in thrombosis of the leg veins.

Embolism is the process in which loose material in the blood-stream lodges in a vessel and impedes the flow beyond it. Usually, the **embolus** is a blood clot that has become dislodged from its original site. A variety of other materials can form emboli, such as air introduced from outside the vascular system (air embolism).

Coronary atherosclerosis

Atherosclerosis of the coronary arteries is the biggest single cause of death, and death in middle age, in the UK and US. It is by far the most frequent cause of myocardial ischaemia, an inadequate blood supply to the heart muscle. The clinical effects depend on the anatomical location, severity and rate of onset of ischaemia.

The ever-pumping myocardium has a high oxygen requirement. Its own blood supply comes from the left and right coronary arteries, which originate in the first part of the aorta (**ascending aorta**), just above the aortic valves (see figure 3.2). Note how these arteries form a crown around the ventricles (hence 'coronary'). Usually, the left coronary artery is the larger; it supplies the more muscular left ventricle and much of the thick muscular interventricular septum (the wall separating the ventricles – see figure 2.8, page 26). The right coronary artery supplies the right ventricle and the posterior part of the heart. A typical arrangement of the main coronary branches is shown in figure 3.2, but there is considerable individual variation and overlap in the areas supplied.

Early events in the development of atherosclerosis are localised changes in the arterial endothelium and the deposition of lipid beneath the endothelium. Chemical changes in the lipid may in turn lead to a series of pathological events in the vessel wall. What initiates the process, how it occurs, and why it progresses more quickly to a severe and complicated form in some people, are not completely known. Certainly, genetic and constitutional factors are important. There are very severe, but relatively rare, forms of atherosclerosis that are due to specific genetically-determined defects in the biochemical processing of cholesterol-containing lipids. Coronary artery disease is common in some families, and rare in others, even allowing for lifestyle differences. Pre-menopausal women are less prone due to the protective effect of **oestrogens** (*female* hormones).

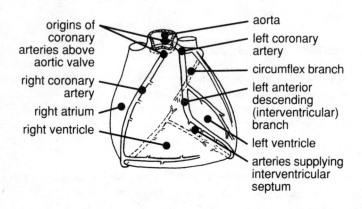

origins of coronary arteries above aortic valve

right coronary artery

right atrium

right ventricle

aorta

left coronary artery

circumflex branch

left anterior descending (interventricular) branch

left ventricle

arteries supplying interventricular septum

Figure 3.2   The coronary arteries

The presence of a high concentration of cholesterol in the blood is strongly correlated with the development of atherosclerosis, and probably does play a causal role in association with other factors. Substantial reduction of a high blood cholesterol by dietary changes and drug treatment, over a long period, does decrease the risk in certain susceptible groups, and may halt progression of plaque in some.

As the atheromatous plaque develops the picture becomes more complicated with the presence of inflammation and repair processes in the arterial wall. Atherosclerosis is usually well advanced when myocardial infarction first occurs, but there may have been no outward signs of heart disease up to that time. Furthermore, the ischaemia leading to infarction is, in most cases, not simply due to the narrowing of the lumen by atherosclerosis but to occlusion of the coronary artery by a thrombus developing rapidly on a disrupted plaque (coronary thrombosis). The factors that can influence the formation of any thrombus are: the state of the vessel wall, the rate and smoothness of blood flow, and the coagulability of the blood (its tendency to clot). In coronary thrombosis all three factors may be important; the endothelium over the plaque may be damaged and favour clot formation, blood flow may be reduced and turbulent in the atherosclerotic artery and increased coagulability may be present before the attack.

There is good evidence that smoking increases the risk of myocardial infarction, possibly by promoting thrombosis and by damaging the endothelium. It also decreases the amount of available oxygen in the blood.

Important risk factors for coronary artery disease are a genetic predisposition, high blood cholesterol, smoking, an abnormally high blood pressure (**hypertension**), obesity and having diabetes mellitus. Some of these are related to dietary risk factors (see chapter eight, page 174).

Myocardial infarction is usually accompanied by severe chest pain which is not relieved by rest and may last several hours. Death sometimes occurs immediately or soon after an attack; the heart stops pumping (**cardiac arrest**), often due to an abnormal heart beat (**arrhythmia**). Cardio-pulmonary resuscitation and rapid access to specialist facilities can often prevent patients dying from dangerous arrhythmias, which may be reversible, or at least manageable. This is one of the main reasons for the proliferation of coronary care units. Other serious events that can occur soon after a coronary thrombosis are cardiac failure (see chapter two, page 31) and shock (due to a severe drop in blood pressure and tissue perfusion).

However, the majority of patients do survive the initial attack relatively unscathed. In the weeks following an uncomplicated myocardial infarction, the myocardium heals and the area of dead muscle is replaced by scar tissue. The ability of the heart to function properly afterwards will depend on what was damaged and to what extent, and on the blood supply available from other vessels to serve the remaining viable heart.

Severe narrowing of a coronary artery can produce recurrent attacks of ischaemic pain without infarction. This is **angina pectoris** (literally, chest pain). Unlike most cases of myocardial infarction, it is not caused by thrombosis. The pain is usually less severe, is brought on by effort and is quickly relieved by rest. The course of angina is variable, sometimes stable for long periods, sometimes progressive; it can even resolve. But the risk of coronary thrombosis is high. Smoking is dangerous.

Atherosclerosis of the aorta and its branches

The aorta rises a short distance above the heart and arches backwards, giving off branches to the head and upper limbs. It then descends in front of the spine to the abdominal cavity to supply the rest of the body. Atherosclerosis sometimes affects the wall of the aorta, particularly the abdominal aorta.

Occasionally the weakened wall of a diseased or defective artery dilates abnormally, forming an **aneurysm**, a sac or bulge in the arterial wall. Atherosclerosis, often assisted by hypertension, is the main cause of **aortic aneurysm** (syphilis was once a common cause). Aneurysms are prone to leak or burst, usually with catastrophic results.

In the abdomen the aorta divides into the arteries supplying the legs. Severe atherosclerosis in these vessels causes muscle ischaemia. This may present as a cramp-like pain in the calf, typically brought on by walking and relieved by rest, a condition known as **intermittent claudicatio**n. The poor blood supply also affects the skin, particularly of the lower leg, which may become hairless and prone to infection. Severe ischaemia eventually leads to necrosis, often starting in the toes. Blackened areas of decay may appear due to infection of the dead tissue by bacteria; this is gangrene.

Stroke

Stroke is a sudden impairment of function due to a blood-vascular event in the brain. It is an important cause of disability and death, especially in the elderly. Most strokes are due to infarction of brain tissue. About ten per cent are due to a haemorrhage within the brain (**intracerebral haemorrhage**).

The brain accounts for nearly a quarter of the body's oxygen consumption. It is rapidly damaged when oxygen and glucose

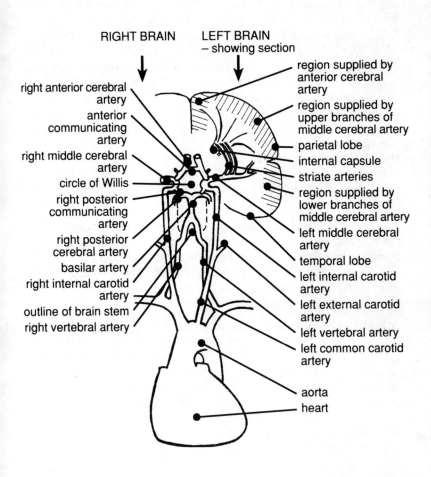

RIGHT BRAIN   LEFT BRAIN
            – showing section

region supplied by anterior cerebral artery

region supplied by upper branches of middle cerebral artery

parietal lobe

internal capsule

striate arteries

region supplied by lower branches of middle cerebral artery

left middle cerebral artery

temporal lobe

left internal carotid artery

left external carotid artery

left vertebral artery

left common carotid artery

aorta

heart

right anterior cerebral artery

anterior communicating artery

right middle cerebral artery

circle of Willis

right posterior communicating artery

right posterior cerebral artery

basilar artery

right internal carotid artery

outline of brain stem

right vertebral artery

Figure 3.3 The brain's blood supply

supplies cease. Not surprisingly, it has an excellent blood supply. Four arteries arise from the large vessels in the chest to supply the head and neck, and in particular the brain (see figure 3.3). They are the left and right carotid arteries, which run up anteriorly, and the left and right vertebral arteries which run up posteriorly either side of the cervical vertebrae. In the upper part of the neck the carotid arteries **bifurcate** (fork into two) into their internal and external branches. Each **internal carotid** then passes into the cranial cavity and bifurcates into the **anterior** and **middle cerebral arteries**, supplying the front and middle parts of the cerebral hemisphere. In the cranium, the left and right vertebral arteries unite to form a short single vessel, **the basilar artery**; these vessels run close to, and supply, the brain stem (the part of the brain connecting the cerebral hemispheres to the spinal cord). The basilar artery then bifurcates to form the left and right **posterior cerebral arteries**, which supply the occipital lobes of the brain.

The three bifurcations that give rise to the six cerebral arteries lie close together at the base of the brain. At this point the systems are linked by **communicating arteries** to form a small arterial ring called the **Circle of Willis**, which provides alternative routes for blood to the cerebral arteries. However, the system is not well formed in some people.

Atherosclerosis in the arteries to the brain occurs mainly at junctions and bends. A common location is the origin of the internal carotid artery. Cerebral (brain) infarcts can be due either to thrombosis at the site of the atherosclerotic lesion or to thromboemboli arising from elsewhere in the cardiovascular system. The thrombus or embolus obstructs blood flow in the cerebral arterial circulation and causes ischaemia in the territory beyond the blockage. Whether or not an infarct occurs, or how extensive it is, depends on, amongst other things, the effectiveness of any alternative (collateral) circulation from other vessels.

The presence of atherosclerosis elsewhere, in the heart for instance, is a risk factor for future development of stroke. Perhaps surprisingly, raised blood cholesterol and smoking have not proved to be prominent risk factors in many studies. A past history of hypertension is important. The rate of development of atherosclerosis in the arteries supplying the brain may be enhanced by a persistently raised blood pressure. Long-standing hypertension also increases the risk of intracerebral haemorrhage. The introduction of effective treatment for hypertension might partly explain the decrease in the occurrence of stroke over the last four decades.

Because of the large number of specialised areas of grey and white matter in the brain, the effect of stroke on function depends very much on the location of the lesion and its size. Blockage of an individual distal branch of a cerebral artery causes a more localised infarct and a more limited clinical effect. For example, a cortical branch of the anterior cerebral artery supplies the *leg* region of the motor and sensory cortex; its occlusion causes weakness or paralysis, and some loss of sensation, in the leg on the side opposite the infarct. Occlusion of the upper branch of the middle cerebral artery affects the lower areas of the motor and sensory cortex and causes paralysis and loss of sensation in the arm and face on the side opposite the lesion.

In the dominant hemisphere the middle cerebral artery supplies the speech centres. Occlusion of its upper cortical branch damages the motor speech area and causes an inability to communicate due to impaired expression (**motor aphasia**), whereas blockage of its lower cortical branch affects the sensory speech area and causes an inability to communicate due to impaired understanding (**sensory aphasia**).

The larger the infarct, the greater will be the range of clinical disability. However, a relatively small lesion deep in the hemisphere can cause extensive impairment. This is because the nerve fibres from different areas of cortex converge into close proximity in a sheath of white matter (the **internal capsule**) before they leave the hemisphere.

Brain damage may continue to progress for a while after occlusion of the artery, and this may be aggravated by particular chemicals released from local tissues. There is a hope that some new medicines under development may be able to limit this extension of damage.

Intracerebral haemorrhage also causes stroke. It is associated with long-standing hypertension which damages small arteries in the brain. Often this involves the **striate branches** of the middle cerebral artery in the region of the internal capsule (see figure 3.3, page 61). The leaking blood cuts through the tracts causing extensive neurological damage.

The onset of stroke is rapid and the effect on function, sometimes the only symptom, is usually maximal within a day. The neurological picture may include various combinations of the following, depending on the location of the lesion: paralysis or weakness on one side (**hemiplegia**, or **monoplegia** if only one limb is affected); sensory loss on one side; loss of vision to one side in both eyes; aphasia if the dominant hemisphere is affected; changes in higher mental functions, sometimes involving mood and personality.

A sudden large intracerebral haemorrhage can produce severe and extensive neurological damage and rapid loss of consciousness; this is classic apoplexy. Headache and vomiting at the onset and change in consciousness are more common after haemorrhage.

The presence of severe atherosclerosis elsewhere, and the absence of hypertension, make infarction a more likely cause. However, in most cases it is difficult to determine the cause with certainty on clinical grounds alone. The differentiation is important if specific therapy is being considered, such as anticoagulants to prevent further thrombosis – this treatment would be disastrous after a cerebral haemorrhage.

About 20 per cent of patients die from their first stroke, and do so mainly in the first month, either from extensive neurological damage or from the complications of being immobile, such as chest infections and pulmonary embolism (see page 66). Of the survivors, two-thirds make a good recovery, achieving functional independence; the remainder are more severely handicapped.

Sometimes patients suffer transient mild strokes which resolve completely within a day. These are called **transient ischaemic attacks** (**TIA**s). They can be due to small emboli from atherosclerotic plaques; a typical site of origin is the carotid bifurcation. Patients having TIAs are at high risk of developing a *completed* stroke with permanent neurological damage. They should be carefully investigated because preventive treatment is sometimes possible.

Hypertension

Hypertension is an arterial blood pressure above an arbitrary reference value. Before proceeding, the reader may wish to review the relevant section in chapter two, page 29.

Blood pressure varies slightly between healthy individuals. It normally increases in response to anxiety, exercise and standing up. After the third decade it also increases gradually with age in many but not all people. Observations on the clinical effects of different blood pressures have provided arbitrary working definitions for hypertension. For people in their third decade it is often defined as a systolic pressure above 140mmHg or a diastolic pressure above 90mmHg. Different values are used for different age groups, to distinguish mild and severe hypertension and to determine the need for drug treatment.

The instrument used to measure blood pressure is a **sphygmomanometer**. The procedure is simple and painless. Anxiety or rushing to the clinic may temporarily raise the pressure. Unless the blood pressure is very high, readings are usually taken on several occasions before labelling the patient with a diagnosis of hypertension.

Persistent hypertension is found in about 15 per cent of the population. In many it is mild and may require observation rather than treatment. Although quite a lot is known about the mechanisms that influence and control blood pressure, the basic cause of persistent hypertension in most patients is unknown. When this is the case the condition is known as **essential** or **primary hypertension**. The muscle fibres in the walls of the small arterial vessels appear to constrict the channels excessively. This offers resistance to blood flow and causes an increase in pressure. Eventually, persistently high pressure causes a structural change in the vessel wall, which tends to further increase the blood pressure. Factors thought to influence the development of essential hypertension include a genetic tendency (it often runs in families), a high salt (sodium chloride) intake, excessive alcohol consumption and obesity.

Hypertension is occasionally due to kidney disease, and very occasionally due to other diseases.

The role of hypertension in stroke has already been mentioned. Long-standing hypertension can also damage the small arterial vessels in the kidney and retina (the layer containing the light-sensitive nerve cells at the back of the eye). Severe hypertension can cause renal failure and produce haemorrhages and other changes in the eye.

Venous thrombosis and pulmonary embolism

Thrombosis sometimes occurs in veins, notably in the deep veins of the leg (**deep vein thrombosis – DVT**). The deep calf muscle (the **soleus**) contains a network of veins which, on contraction of the muscle, pump venous blood up the leg. Prolonged immobility can produce stagnation of blood in the deep leg veins and a risk of thrombosis. Deep vein thrombosis is a common complication in elderly patients immobilised by stroke or fractured hip. It sometimes occurs after myocardial infarction and surgical operations, usually within two weeks. A DVT may present as a painful or swollen leg, or may be symptomless. The condition is potentially dangerous.

The deep vein thrombus is often fragile. Sometimes it breaks away, travels in the venous blood stream, passes through the right side of the heart and then lodges in the pulmonary arteries (**pulmonary embolism**). The effect depends on the size of the thrombus and the state of the patient. A very large thrombus can completely obstruct the pulmonary arteries and cause sudden death. Smaller thromboemboli may produce localised areas of lung infarction, which may cause chest pain or the coughing of blood (**haemoptysis**). Pulmonary embolism can present in a number of different ways. Small emboli are sometimes symptomless.

Deep vein thrombosis must be distinguished from the inflammation and thrombosis that sometimes occurs in the more superficial veins under the skin. In the latter condition (**thrombophlebitis**) the clot is firmly adherent to the inflamed vein wall and rarely causes pulmonary embolism.

Tumours and cancer

Introduction

A **tumour** (or **neoplasm**) is an abnormal swelling due to a new growth of cells which has no useful function.

Tumours are benign or malignant. **Benign tumours** expand locally and sometimes cause pressure on neighbouring structures but they do not usually extend beyond the tissue boundary. Their cells resemble those of the tissue of origin. Some benign tumours occasionally change into malignant tumours.

Malignant tumours contain abnormal cells which proliferate, invade and spread beyond their tissue of origin without regard for normal constraints and controls. **Cancer** is the term applied to all diseases characterised by malignant cell growth. Cancerous lesions are mostly tumours, but they can present in other ways. For example, **leukaemia** is a diffuse proliferation of malignant white blood cells.

Malignant cells spread from their site of origin by destroying and invading adjacent tissues and boundaries, by infiltrating lymphatic vessels and lymph nodes, and via the blood stream to distant tissues and organs. The tumour at the site of origin is the **primary tumour**. Its offshoots seeding and growing at distant sites are called **secondary tumours** or **metastases**. Lung, liver, bone and brain are typical sites for metastases, the predilection depending on the nature of the primary tumour.

Cancer is the second greatest cause of death in western civilisation. It is responsible for a quarter of all deaths in the UK and US. In these countries major malignancies are carcinomas of the lung, large bowel, breast and prostate; together they account for 50 per cent of all cancer deaths.

Tumour nomenclature and classification

Precise classification of the nature and the extent of spread of a tumour is essential for an accurate assessment of the outlook for the patient and the selection of appropriate treatment.

Technical terms abound, they are necessary for accurate communication, but to illustrate the principles we need only consider a few.

The suffix **-oma** means tumour. Used alone or as a suffix the terms carcinoma and sarcoma (see below) refer to malignant tumours. Sometimes the first part of the name indicates the particular tissue of origin. Thus, a **lipoma** is a benign tumour of fat cells (commonly seen as a discrete skin-covered fatty lump), and a **liposarcoma** is its very rare malignant counterpart. Similarly, **osteoma** and **osteosarcoma** are respectively benign and malignant forms of bone tumour. Unfortunately, the nomenclature is not entirely consistent; for instance, leukaemia, lymphoma and melanoma are malignant.

A **carcinoma** is a malignant tumour originating from epithelium, the tissue covering the internal and external surfaces of the body, including the linings of various ducts. It is the commonest type of malignancy, the type most often responsible for cancer of the lung, breast, bowel, stomach, liver, pancreas, womb and prostate. **Sarcomas** are relatively rare. They arise from tissues of mesodermal origin that lie beneath the epithelia, such as bone, cartilage and muscle.

Under the microscope, malignant tumours have characteristic features that distinguish them from benign tumours. They vary in the extent to which their microscopic appearance resembles that of the tissue of origin. When the resemblance is close the tumour is said to be **well differentiated**, and when poor it is **poorly differentiated**. Sometimes tumours are so poorly differentiated that all resemblance to the original tissue is lost; these are **anaplastic** tumours. Classification based on the degree of differentiation is known as **grading**. As a general rule, the more poorly differentiated the tumour, the more aggressive and invasive it is likely to be.

Another type of classification, known as **staging**, describes tumour spread. For example, the **TNM system** uses numbers to define the extent of infiltration of the primary tumour (**T**), extent of spread to the lymph nodes (**N**) and the presence of metastases (**M**).

A simple but important point is that tumour nomenclature generally refers to the site of origin. Thus, the term 'carcinoma of the lung' indicates that the primary tumour is in the lung, but there may also be secondary deposits of the tumour in other organs.

The cause of cancer

Thanks to many decades of painstaking research we now know enough about the cause of cancer, and how it develops, to make some important general statements. Much of the detail still awaits discovery. The simplified account that follows aims to provide an outline of current thinking.

Normally, many mechanisms operate in concert to regulate the growth, specialisation, proliferation, mobility, orientation and location of cells in a tissue. They involve chemical signals within and between cells and feed-back control systems. A relatively small number of key genes are responsible for the overall control of these operations. They regulate the societal behaviour of the cell. Cancer occurs when they fail to function normally due to faults in chromosome DNA structure. Conversion to the malignant state (**transformation**) seems to require the presence in the cell of at least two, probably more, defective genes. Some of these genes produce cancer by means of their unbridled over-activity (**oncogenes**), others do it by switching off their normal cancer-suppressing activity (**onco-suppressor genes**). Many of these effects occur in conjunction with abnormalities of chromosome structure and production commonly seen in malignant cells.

The tendency of some cancers to run in families can be due to the inheritance of a faulty gene, but the disease will not appear until the accumulation of faulty genetic material reaches some critical combination or level in a particular cell. Humans acquire most of their cancer-associated genetic faults during their lifetime. Cancer occurs most frequently in the middle-aged and elderly. Those who start off with inherited faults are at greater risk and will tend to get the disease earlier than those without.

There are other biological factors that increase or decrease susceptibility to cancer. For example, cells normally have a certain capacity to repair faults in DNA structure. When this mechanism is defective (which is rare) the risk of cancer is higher. The immune system recognises and attacks some cancer cells. People with deficient immune responses are sometimes more prone to particular types of cancer.

Agents known as **carcinogens** (cancer producing substances), which may be particular chemicals or forms of radiation, are largely responsible for the changes in DNA structure that lead to malignancy. They produce a chemical change in a segment of the DNA molecule, which is misread when the cell divides. This causes substitution of the wrong DNA base (see chapter two, page 16) and perpetuation of a message error in subsequent cell divisions. Many chemical carcinogens are converted into their active form by metabolism in the body. The chemical carcinogens in tobacco smoke are responsible for most cases of lung cancer. Some viruses may act as carcinogens by introducing new genetic material into the cell. They certainly play a role in the development of some tumours (see page 83), but their importance as causative agents in the commoner cancers of developed countries is uncertain. The important point is that the majority of human cancers appear to be due to external agents and are therefore potentially preventable.

The primary tumour arises from a single malignant cell. Initially the cells probably multiply regularly but later the rate of growth of the tumour progressively slows. This is because an increasingly larger proportion of the cells stop dividing and enter a prolonged resting phase, probably due to lack of oxygen and blood supply. Sometimes the deeper cells die, producing an area of necrosis in the tumour. Large tumours may take many months to double in size. Cells in the resting phase can become active again. They may do so if most, but not all, of the tumour mass is removed, whether by surgical or medical treatment. Many of the medical treatments are more effective against actively dividing cells.

Malignant cells often produce new genetic variants, with even more genetic faults. The more aggressive cells tend to dominate. Consequently, the nature of the tumour may change with time, tending to become more malignant. This may occur in the metastases independently of the primary tumour.

The treatment protocol requires careful consideration of these and many other factors.

Some clinical aspects of cancer

There are many forms of cancer and each has its own peculiarities and problems. The course of a particular cancer and its likely response to treatment depend on the type of tumour and its grading, the anatomical location of the primary lesion and the extent of spread to distant sites.

Carcinomas usually form solid tumours. When these are near the surface of the body and easily accessible, such as in the skin or breast, they may be seen or felt as a discrete lump. However, even the smallest detectable tumour contains many millions of cells. Tumours of the internal organs are usually much larger before they cause obvious symptoms and make themselves known. Some carcinomas take the form of an ulcer, an erosion or crater-like area, rather than a lump.

Local invasion and erosion of small blood vessels causes bleeding. Thus, carcinomas of the lung, large bowel and kidney may reveal themselves by the presence of blood in the sputum, faeces and urine respectively. Similarly, abnormal bleeding from the vagina might signify the presence of a uterine (womb) tumour. Bleeding is a non-specific symptom and it can be due to many other, non-malignant, conditions.

A change in the function of one of the body's tubes or channels can be an early symptom when a tumour obstructs it from within, or compresses it from without. A carcinoma of the large bowel may extend into the lumen and interfere with the passage of bowel contents. This may present as an unexplained change in bowel habit or, in the case of a complete blockage, as an **intestinal obstruction**, a condition characterised by an inability to pass faeces and wind (**flatus**), swelling of the abdomen and vomiting. A carcinoma of the prostate may compress the urethra and prevent the passage of urine from the bladder (as can benign enlargement of the prostate, a common condition in older men). Malignant tumours in the liver and in the region of the bile channels may interfere with the circulation of bile and cause jaundice. A carcinoma of the bronchus can obstruct air flow in the lung.

Metastases produce effects too, but they can be symptomless. Secondary deposits in bone sometimes cause pain. Brain metastases can produce localised neurological abnormalities, personality changes or fits.

Contrary to popular belief, pain is not a universal feature of cancer. Particular causes of pain are: direct invasion and compression of nerves by the tumour, the stretching of organs by large deposits, and bone pain due to the weakening effect of some bone metastases (sometimes fractures occur).

Unexplained weight loss and **anorexia** (loss of appetite) are later features of many cancers. Sometimes the wasting is extreme and also involves the muscles. This generally weakened and wasted state is called **cachexia**. Its cause is not entirely clear but the tumour appears to alter the metabolism of the body.

These are just a few of the effects produced by malignant tumours. Many of the symptoms are non-specific and can occur in other conditions.

Lung cancer

Carcinoma of the bronchus (bronchial carcinoma) is by far the commonest form of lung cancer, and the commonest lethal cancer in the UK and US. It occurs most frequently between the ages of 45 and 75 years. The tumour arises from the epithelium lining the air passages, particularly the larger bronchi. There are different types of bronchial carcinoma, with different characteristics, courses and problems.

Smoking is the most important cause of carcinoma of the bronchus. The evidence is overwhelming. The tar component of tobacco smoke contains potent carcinogens, the more inhaled the greater the risk of cancer.

Typical early clinical manifestations of bronchial carcinoma are persistent cough, coughing blood (**haemoptysis**) and recurrent lung infection. Sometimes the primary tumour obstructs air flow and fluid drainage in a bronchus. The pulmonary blood capillaries absorb the trapped air, causing the surrounding area of lung to collapse; fluid accumulates beyond the obstruction and infection sets in. Recurrent localised lung infection is a typical early feature of tumours obstructing the larger proximal branches of the bronchial tree. Tumours nearer the periphery of the lung are less likely to present in this way and may spread further before symptoms become obvious.

Depending on its location, direct spread of the tumour within the chest may affect a variety of structures, such as nerves, air passages, large blood vessels, the diaphragm and the chest wall. Lymphatic spread leads to invasion and enlargement of lymph nodes, particularly those deep in the chest. Common sites for metastases are brain, liver and bone.

Some bronchial carcinomas release chemicals, including hormones, which have strange and often serious effects on other parts of the body. Just one example is an inappropriate release of an antidiuretic hormone (ADH) which leads to abnormal retention of water and dilution of the blood.

For patients with very malignant anaplastic forms of bronchial carcinoma the outlook is poor. Metastases are almost always present at the time of diagnosis, when life expectancy without treatment is generally about three months. With treatment this can sometimes be extended to about one year. On the other hand, appropriate surgery for a favourably located well-differentiated tumour with limited spread and no detectable metastases provides a cure in some 50 per cent of patients, as measured by survival to 5 years after treatment. Generally, however, cancer of the lung has a bad prognosis.

Cancer of the large bowel

The lumen of the large bowel is lined with an epithelium which secretes substances such as mucus onto the surface. A benign tumour of this epithelium is known as an **adenoma**. The large bowel adenoma takes the form of a **polyp**, a knob of tissue protruding from the surface into the lumen. An **adenocarcinoma**, the corresponding malignant tumour, usually arises in a pre-existing benign adenoma.

Adenocarcinoma of the large bowel, including the rectum, is a relatively common cancer in men and women. It occurs mainly after the age of 40 years and its frequency of occurrence continues to increase into the seventh decade.

A progressive accumulation of genetic faults appears to be

responsible for the transition from normal epithelial cell to benign adenoma and later, usually after some years, from adenoma to malignant adenocarcinoma. Some people inherit cancer-susceptibility genes which may shorten the time scale to the appearance of malignancy. A few unfortunate people suffer from a rare but strongly inherited disorder in which vast numbers of intestinal polyps appear at adolescence; without preventive treatment (surgical) they are very liable to develop cancer of the bowel in early adult life. The evidence suggests that exposure of the bowel to carcinogens during a person's lifetime is probably the most important causative factor in adenocarcinoma of the large bowel. There is less certainty about which carcinogens are responsible but certain types of diet and cooking process might be important.

Some of the clinical effects of bowel cancer were mentioned earlier. Not surprisingly, given the direct connection of the portal vein, metastases occur most commonly in the liver.

Overall, after modern treatment for large bowel cancer about 50 per cent of patients are still alive at five and ten years, and are therefore assumed to be cured. The survival rate is better than this when the carcinoma is confined to a small region of bowel wall, and worse if it has spread to the lymph nodes and elsewhere.

Breast cancer

Lumps commonly occur in the female breast. Most are not malignant, nor potentially malignant. All are a cause for concern because the distinction between benign and malignant tumours by external manual examination of the breast alone is often unreliable, even in the hands of trained professionals. Currently, breast cancer affects about eight per cent of women in the UK and US.

The mature female breast comprises the milk-forming apparatus and the fibrous and fatty tissues which support and protect it. Numerous milk-forming units drain into small ducts which link up to form fewer and larger ducts which eventually emerge at the nipple. The form and function of this tissue is strongly influenced by the levels of several circulating female hormones. The most obvious changes occur during pregnancy and nursing (feeding a baby at the breast). Changes also occur during the normal monthly menstrual cycle. This is often noticeable just before a period when the breasts may become enlarged and tender due to proliferation of milk-gland tissue. Between the age of 30 years and menopause (when the periods stop, at about 50 years) the process may become more noticeable with the development of a diffuse lumpiness in the breasts, a common benign condition known as **fibrocystic change**.

Carcinoma of the breast usually arises from the epithelial cells lining the small ducts. It occurs mainly after 40 years of age, and particularly after the menopause. Women with a family history of breast cancer (e.g. mother, sister) are at a slightly greater risk of developing the disease. In a few families the inherited genetic risk is higher, and the disease tends to appear earlier.

Female hormones can influence the development of breast cancer. The cells of many breast carcinomas have special oestrogen receptor molecules on their surface. Oestrogens stimulate the growth of these cells. The blockage of this effect by specific drugs is proving to be an effective form of treatment. A long reproductive life (i.e. the number of years from first to last period), no pregnancies or a late age at first pregnancy slightly increase the risk of breast cancer. There have been differences of opinion over the effect of the oral contraceptive pill on the risk of developing breast cancer, but present evidence suggests that the low dose forms are unlikely to increase the risk much, if at all.

Studies of the occurrence of breast cancer in migrant populations suggest that environmental influences are important. The main causative agents have not yet been identified with certainty, but diet may be important (see chapter eight, page 177).

A carcinoma of the breast may take a matter of years to grow into a **palpable** (easily felt) tumour. It may then be the size of a small grape and contain more than a thousand million cells. Even at this stage malignant cells may have reached the local lymph nodes, in the armpit (**axilla**) for example, or spread to other sites. This is less likely with small tumours. Microscopic examination of surgically removed axillary lymph nodes is often important for the determination of prognosis and treatment. If the nodes contain malignant cells there are more likely to be metastases at distant sites such as bone (e.g. spine), lung or liver, although they may not become apparent until months or years later.

The prognosis depends largely on the stage of the tumour at the time of the first treatment. The newer X-ray techniques for screening the breast (**mammography**) pick up tumours at an earlier stage than with manual examination alone and there is already evidence that they are improving the outlook for women with this disease. For bowel cancer a five year survival after treatment often equates with a cure. The same is not true for breast cancer which can recur many years after apparently successful treatment. Survival to 20 years without a recurrence may approximate to a cure. Complete surgical removal of a small favourably located carcinoma confined to breast tissue with no lymph node involvement offers good prospects; probably more than 75 per cent of patients in this category will still be alive ten years later. Earlier detection may further improve the prognosis. The survival rate is lower when the lymph nodes are involved. The treatment of breast cancer has changed considerably in recent years, but there is not yet a complete consensus of opinion. Treatment may involve surgery, radiotherapy or chemotherapy, or a combination of these, depending on the stage of the disease. Advances are being made and it is reasonable to expect that the prognosis of breast cancer will continue to improve. Early detection and prompt and adequate surgical removal are important (also see chapters eight and nine, pages 191 and 211).

Concluding remarks

The number of deaths from a particular cancer in a given period does not necessarily reflect the frequency of occurrence of that cancer. For anaplastic forms of bronchial carcinoma the figures are close because the disease is often fatal. Some forms of skin cancer are very common but they are eminently treatable and the death rate due to them is very low. A rarer type of skin cancer, the malignant melanoma, has a higher mortality. Earlier detection, better treatment and changing occurrence all influence subsequent mortality figures for individual cancers, so careful interpretation is required.

Cancer also occurs in children but it is comparatively rare. Its forms are diverse and differ considerably from those of adult cancers. Certain types of childhood **leukaemia** (proliferation of malignant white blood cells) respond well to modern drug therapy.

Although occurrence varies both between and within countries, on the whole the same types of cancer tend to dominate in the different western industrialised societies. Other parts of the world have different cancer problems. For instance, carcinomas of the oesophagus and liver are especially common in China. Carcinoma of the stomach is much more common in Japan than in the West, while breast cancer is less common. Environmental factors are important in the development of many cancers. Other aspects of cancer are dealt with in chapters eight and nine.

Infection

Introduction

The world around us is bristling with tiny creatures invisible to the naked eye. They are the **micro-organisms** such as bacteria and viruses. Some of them find the environment of the human body favourable for their nourishment, succour and reproduction. Many live in harmony with us. They colonise our body surfaces, orifices and bowel, and some even live in our cells. Some are positively beneficial. Occasionally, micro-organisms carry out their activities at the expense of the person harbouring them (the **host**) and may then be harmful and cause disease. **Infection** is the invasion of the body by disease-causing (**pathogenic**) micro-organisms, commonly known as germs. The severity and outcome of an infection depend on the aggressiveness of the micro-organism and the effectiveness of the host's defences.

Infection is still a major cause of death and suffering in the underdeveloped world. Until the twentieth century it was also the main cause of death and a short life span in western industrialised countries. Improvements in sanitation, hygiene, living conditions and nutrition, and the introduction of immunisation and effective medical treatments have dramatically reduced the incidence and effects of serious infections. Modern technology and the life-styles and trappings of developed societies encourage the emergence of different patterns of infection.

Inflammation

A most important response of a tissue to infection or injury is **inflammation**. It is easily seen in the skin following stings and scratches. It consists of an increased blood flow to the area followed by leakage of fluid from small blood vessels into the tissue spaces. The result is localised redness, warmth and swelling, and often pain and tenderness. The inflammatory reaction localises and lessens the effect of infection. It also focuses the activities of the white blood cells and antibodies, which attempt to destroy invading micro-organisms.

Inflammation may occur suddenly and last from a few hours to a few weeks (**acute**) or may be more protracted (**chronic**). Its characteristics depend on many factors such as the particular type of micro-organism or injurious agent involved, the nature of the tissue or organ affected and the state of health of the patient. The inflammatory reaction sometimes results in permanent tissue damage.

In medical terminology the suffix **-itis** denotes inflammation. Thus, inflammation of the bronchial tubes, heart, liver and kidney is **bronchitis**, **carditis**, **hepatitis** and **nephritis** respectively. Inflammation of the brain is **encephalitis** and that of the membranes covering it is **meningitis**. **Pneumonia** is an exception, being the term for an inflammatory reaction in the lung in which fluid accumulates in the gas-exchange units (alveoli).

Bacteria

Bacteria are cells, smaller than human cells. Many can survive in both living and non-living (e.g. food, water, soil) environments. They reproduce by splitting in half to form two identical daughter cells. Bacteria differ from human cells in a number of ways, such as in the structure and composition of the cell

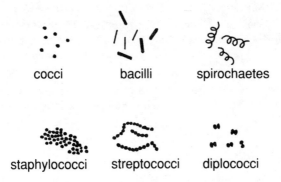

Figure 3.4 Types of bacteria

wall and in some aspects of their metabolism. They have just one chromosome and no nuclear membrane. The differences are important in the search for new antibiotics that can attack pathogenic bacteria without harming us.

We can distinguish different types of bacteria by their shape (see figure 3.4) and many other properties. The **coccus** is spherical, the **bacillus** is rod-like and the **spirochaete** is spiral. Table 3.1 lists just a few of the diseases that bacteria can cause. Each particular type of bacterium has a name. For instance, the bacillus causing typhoid fever is known as **Salmonella typhi**. The second part of the name indicates the particular sub-group (species) of Salmonella. **Salmonella typhimurium** is a different species; it is one of a number of bacteria responsible for food poisoning. Species can be further sub-divided into strains. Some strains cause more severe infections than others.

Bacteria may cause inflammation and tissue damage near their point of entry to the body or at more distant sites. For instance, the coccus known as **Neisseria meningitidis** invades the body through the nose and throat but finds its way to the membranes covering the brain (**meninges**) where it causes meningitis (often called meningococcal meningitis

Disease	Typical features
caused by cocci:	
Meningococcal meningitis	acute inflammation of membranes covering brain; fever, headache, neck stiffness; sometimes has serious complications
Pneumococcal pneumonia	acute inflammation of lung; fever, often chest pain at early stage
Gonorrhoea	inflammation of genital tract; discharge from urethra in men
caused by bacilli (rods):	
Diphtheria	severe sore throat, sometimes airway obstruction; toxin from bacterium causes inflammation of heart muscle
Whooping cough	severe coughing bouts; can cause pneumonia and permanent lung damage
Tuberculosis	damaging chronic inflammation of lung; can affect many organs
Typhoid fever	fever; ulceration of small bowel
caused by a spirochaete:	
Syphilis	several stages: local genital lesions first, then generalised infection and rash; late effects include damage to heart, aorta and nervous system

Table 3.1 Some infectious diseases caused by bacteria

when caused by this organism). Some bacteria produce **toxins** (poisonous substances) and some cause allergic reactions. Let us enlarge by reference to just three particular bacteria: Staphylococcus aureus, Streptococcus pyogenes and Clostridium tetani.

Staphylococci are cocci that congregate in clusters (see figure 3.4). **Staphylococcus aureus** is a pus-forming (pyogenic) species. It can cause skin infections (e.g. boils), abscesses (collections of pus) in many parts of the body, wound infections, infection of the blood stream (septicaemia) and a dangerous form of pneumonia. It is an important cause of infection in hospitals. To make matters worse some strains of Staphylococcus aureus have become resistant to most antibiotics.

Streptococci are cocci that assemble in chains (see figure 3.4). **Streptococcus pyogenes** is also pyogenic and can cause skin infections (**impetigo**, **erysipelas**) and sore throats. It can also cause more widespread effects by mechanisms other than direct invasion of the tissues. Sometimes streptococci infecting the throat produce a toxin which causes a diffuse bright red skin rash (scarlet fever). Occasionally, streptococcal sore throats lead to allergic reactions affecting the heart and joints (rheumatic fever) or the kidney (nephritis).

The bacillus known as **Clostridium tetani** causes **tetanus** (lock-jaw), a life-threatening disease in which the muscles of the jaw, face, neck and trunk go into severe spasm. The bacillus is present in excreta and soil and may enter the skin during injury. It thrives in dirty wounds but remains localised near the site of entry. It produces its effect by releasing a toxin which acts on motor neurons in the spinal cord, the nerve cells sending signals to the muscles.

Viruses

Unlike the bacterium, the virus is so small it cannot be seen with an ordinary (light) microscope. It consists primarily of nucleic acid, either DNA or RNA, surrounded by a protein coat. The nucleic acid contains the information necessary for reproduction but in order to replicate, that is to make molecular copies of itself, the virus must gain access to a living cell and usurp its biochemical machinery and nutrients. Viral replication damages and eventually kills the host cell. The newly-formed viruses infect other cells. Some cells produce a special protein called **interferon** which helps to protect healthy cells from virus infection. The overall clinical effect depends on the extent of tissue damage. The infection may be so limited that it causes no obvious symptoms. Some of the diseases that viruses can cause are listed in table 3.2.

RNA viruses replicate in the cytoplasm of the cell. DNA viruses replicate in the nucleus and can also merge with human DNA. They may remain dormant in living cells for years. The herpes group of viruses, which are responsible for cold sores,

Disease	Typical features
caused by RNA viruses:	
Influenza	fever, aches and pains, nausea, vomiting, cough; post-flu depression
Measles	cold-like symptoms followed by red rash; occasional complications, such as pneumonia
Rubella (German measles)	usually a mild disease; pink rash; dangerous in early pregnancy – can cause heart, brain and eye defects in fetus
Poliomyelitis	fever, headache, neck and back stiffness; attacks neurons supplying muscles; sometimes causes permanent paralysis, e.g. in legs
Hepatitis A	acute inflammation of liver; abdominal pain and jaundice; recovery usual
caused by DNA viruses:	
Chicken pox	itchy skin rash with crops of small blisters containing infectious fluid or pus. Virus stays in body for rest of life
Shingles	re-activation of chicken pox virus in later life, especially in elderly; pain and typical localised rash on one side of body
Genital herpes	caused by virus called Herpes simplex (which also causes cold sores); eruptions on external genitalia; attacks may recur
Hepatitis B	clinically similar to hepatitis A except that infection may become chronic and cause permanent liver damage; carcinoma of liver sometimes associated with chronic hepatitis B
caused by retrovirus:	
AIDS	caused by human immunodeficiency virus (HIV); slowly damages immune system, leaving patient susceptible to other infections (see text)

Table 3.2 Some infectious diseases caused by viruses

genital herpes, chicken pox and shingles stay with us for life. They may become active under certain circumstances and then produce ill effects. Perhaps not surprisingly, DNA viruses are thought to play a role in the development of some cancers. Chronic hepatitis B virus infection plays an important role in the development of liver cancer, which is common in Southeast Asia and Africa. The human papilloma virus (HPV) may be one of the causative factors in carcinoma of the cervix and penis.

The retrovirus, one variety of which causes AIDS, is a special type of RNA virus. It has an enzyme which produces in the host cell a DNA copy of its RNA message. The DNA copy can then merge with human genetic material.

Viruses have a predilection for particular tissues. Some produce their main effects near their point of entry to the body. The common cold and influenza viruses attack cells lining the air passages. Others need to spread within the body to find their target cells. For instance, hepatitis A and B viruses produce little effect at their points of entry but specifically invade and damage liver cells.

Other organisms

Micro-organisms other than bacteria and viruses also cause disease. **Plasmodium** is the protozoan (single-cell animal) responsible for **malaria**, one of the world's most important infections. **Chlamydiae** (singular, chlamydia) resemble bacteria in some respects and, like viruses, they live inside cells. They are responsible for a variety of diseases including **trachoma** (an important eye disease in Africa and Asia), respiratory tract infections and a sexually-transmitted disease resembling gonorrhoea. **Fungus** infections are common but usually mild and superficial; well known examples are **thrush** and **ringworm**.

Animals consisting of more than one cell (**metazoa**) can also live on or invade the body (**infestation**). **Mites** are tiny spider-like creatures. One particular type is responsible for scabies, a contagious and extremely itchy skin infestation. **Lice** are small wingless blood-sucking insects which can infest the body surface and cause skin irritation. Some mites and lice transmit pathogenic micro-organisms to man. There are many types of worm that use the human body as part of their life cycle and some cause serious disease, particularly in the tropics.

Spread of infection

A **communicable disease** is one that passes from person to person. The transfer of infection generally occurs during a particular phase of the illness. Diseases may be spread by direct contact (e.g. sexually transmitted diseases such as syphilis, gonorrhoea and HIV infection), by eating or drinking food or water contaminated with faecal material (e.g. typhoid, hepatitis A, poliomyelitis) or by inhaling infected airborne droplets from coughs and sneezes (e.g. colds, influenza, measles, rubella, chicken pox, diphtheria, whooping cough, meningococcal meningitis, tuberculosis). Another important means of spreading disease is the use of contaminated needles by drug abusers (hepatitis B, HIV). Some people can harbour pathogenic micro-organisms for long periods without becoming ill, but they may be a source of infection to others or even to themselves at a later date. For instance, Staphylococcus aureus residing in the nose can be the cause of wound infection after surgery.

A pathogenic micro-organism risks extinction if it kills its main host too rapidly and too often. A disease due to an organism that has been present in a population for a long time tends to be of a less severe nature. With the passage of time less aggressive variants of the organism may emerge and the affected population may develop a degree of resistance to the infection. Acute diseases with high mortality rates sometimes occur when man is an incidental and occasional rather than an essential part of the micro-organism's life cycle (e.g. rabies, Ebola disease).

The ease with which micro-organisms spread and infect varies considerably. Whooping cough, chicken pox and measles are examples of highly infectious diseases. An **epidemic** is the simultaneous outbreak of an infection in many people in a community or country; if it spreads worldwide it becomes a **pandemic**. **Influenza epidemics** of mild to moderate severity occur most winters. Because the virus frequently changes its form, the immunity gained after one attack does not necessarily confer protection during subsequent epidemics. Very occasionally a new and very aggressive strain of influenza virus emerges to which the human population has little immunity. The resulting pandemic can be devastating; that of 1918 accounted for more than 20 million deaths.

Animals are the main host of some organisms that can cause disease in man (e.g. rabies). Some creatures act as essential intermediary carriers of infection. For example, the mosquito transfers the yellow fever virus from monkey to human and from human to human. It also transmits the malarial parasite (Plasmodium) from person to person.

Some germs can survive in dust and dried secretions or on contaminated materials and instruments, which may act as sources of infection (e.g. Staphylococcus aureus, tuberculosis bacillus, hepatitis B virus).

Developed countries may have fewer serious problems with infectious diseases but there is no room for complacency. The increased speed and freedom of international travel facilitates the acquisition and spread of infection. The increasing resistance of micro-organisms to drug therapy is a worldwide problem. The waning of immunisation in the UK has led to a resurgence of diseases such as whooping cough. Sexual lifestyles and intravenous drug abuse practices influence the spread of HIV and other infections. Food poisoning is still a problem. The bacillus **Legionella** breeds in stagnant water in plumbing and air conditioning systems; inhalation of infected water droplets can cause a form of pneumonia (**Legionnaires' disease**). The message is that changes in our lifestyle patterns also cause changes in the ecology of pathogenic micro-organisms, sometimes to our disadvantage.

First lines of defence

Like all forms of life, micro-organisms take advantage of opportunity. A damaged or inefficient defence system renders the host more susceptible to serious disease from infection, even by micro-organisms that are not normally pathogenic in healthy individuals.

Healthy intact skin, assisted by its normally harmless residential bacteria, is an excellent barrier to germs. Dirt, wounds, burns and some skin disorders increase the risk of infection. Even small cracks and abrasions may be sufficient to allow access to organisms such as Staphylococcus aureus and hepatitis B virus, when handling contaminated materials for instance.

The epithelia of the digestive and respiratory tracts produce mucus and other substances to ward off unwanted organisms. The constant flow of tears, saliva and urine is important in preventing infection of the eyes, mouth and urinary tract respectively. Similarly, the lowest parts of the respiratory tract are normally kept virtually sterile by the constant upward flow of mucus, and the odd cough, which carry debris and organisms towards the throat for clearance. Structural damage or obstruction in the respiratory and renal tracts can impair flow, cause stagnation of fluid and leave surfaces vulnerable. Under these conditions micro-organisms, even some that are normally harmless in other parts of the body, are able to multiply and cause infection. Influenza sometimes damages the epithelium of the lower respiratory tract leaving it vulnerable to severe bacterial infection. In chronic bronchitis there is over-production of bronchial mucus and a tendency to chest infections, which further exacerbate the condition.

The internal defence systems

When micro-organisms invade the tissues the next line of defence comes into operation. It involves inflammation and specialised cells. **Phagocytes** are cells that can engulf and destroy bacteria. **Polymorphs** are phagocytic white blood cells. They migrate from the blood stream to sites of acute inflammation to participate in the battle. Polymorphs are short-lived and require continuous replenishment from the bone marrow. Pus, the yellowish or greenish fluid found in boils and abscesses, is largely an accumulation of the remains of dead polymorphs. A longer-lived phagocyte, the **macrophage**, lurks in the tissues and participates in chronic inflammatory reactions associated with certain infections, such as tuberculosis, leprosy and syphilis. So-called **natural killer cells** attack and destroy cells infected by viruses.

The most specific reaction to infection is the **immune response**, which is the remit of special cells called **lymphocytes**. It is the mechanism by which a single exposure to an infectious organism, such as measles virus, leads to long-standing immunity to subsequent infection by the same agent. It is the basis of immunisation (see chapter eight, page 186). Lymphocytes circulate in the blood (they are another type of white cell) and in the lymphatic system. They are abundant in special **lymphoid tissues** such as the **lymph nodes**, **spleen** and **tonsils**. There are two main types, B- and T-lymphocytes.

B-lymphocytes are responsible for the production of **antibodies**, specific proteins capable of recognising and locking onto foreign molecular structures (**antigens**), such as part of a bacterial cell wall. An antigen is a substance that stimulates the production of antibodies towards its own molecular structure. Antibodies are also known as **immunoglobulins**. Some circulate in plasma and into the tissues. Other types are present in the digestive, respiratory and renal tracts where they help protect against invasion by micro-organisms. Antibodies are important in the fight against pathogenic bacteria and they can neutralise the effects of bacterial toxins (e.g. tetanus toxin).

The surface of the **T-lymphocyte** contains specific receptors, immunoglobulin-like molecules, which enable it to lock onto a cell with a particular type of antigen on its surface. Thus, T-lymphocytes can recognise, attack and kill infected cells. Others regulate the immune response. T-lymphocytes combat infections caused by viruses, fungi, protozoa and certain bacteria (e.g. tuberculosis). They participate in the chronic inflammatory reaction.

When a new antigen appears in the body the immune system takes a few days to process the information and produce new lymphocytes capable of making specific immunoglobulins. Subsequent exposure causes a more rapid response because some lymphocytes still hold the memory of the relevant immunoglobulin structures and they can proliferate immediately and provide protection. This system provides immunity to re-infection from many infectious diseases including whooping cough, diphtheria, measles and poliomyelitis. The common cold recurs frequently because there are hundreds of variant common cold viruses and new antibodies must be made each time to match the different molecular structures. The problem of influenza was mentioned earlier on page 84.

The various components of the internal defence system interact closely and some control or modify the activities of others. Infections occur more frequently and are of greater severity when there are faults in the system. Several rare inherited defects are known. Acquired (i.e. non-inherited) conditions associated with frequent infection include AIDS (see page 91), failure to make new white cells (which is sometimes due to taking certain drugs), and leukaemia (where abnormal white cells are present in the blood). The higher concentration of glucose in the tissues of people with diabetes renders them more liable to bacterial and fungal infections (e.g. boils, thrush).

The effects of infection

The clinical features of infection are due to the local effects on the target tissues and general effects on the body (e.g. fever). The destructive activities of invading micro-organisms and the accompanying inflammation cause the local tissue damage. Bacterial toxins and allergic reactions may also cause damage in tissues other than those directly invaded by the organism. The inflammatory reaction varies considerably depending on the micro-organism and the tissue involved. The **acute** response in the common cold, for instance, consists of swelling of the membranes lining the upper air passages and a profuse watery discharge, giving rise to a stuffy and runny nose. Pyogenic bacteria cause purulent (pussy) inflammation; infection by Staphylococcus aureus produces localised collections of pus (**abscesses**) in the affected tissues. Infection of a duct in the skin (e.g. hair follicle) causes the form of abscess known as a boil. Eventually, an abscess may discharge its contents onto a surface and drain the unwanted materials.

Chronic inflammation, which may follow unresolved acute inflammation or arise from particular infections (e.g. tuberculosis), tends to cause more permanent tissue damage and scar formation. Infection and inflammation, acute or chronic, can affect the function of the afflicted tissue. This may have serious consequences when an important organ is involved.

There is a time lapse (**incubation period**) between the exposure to infection and the appearance of clinical symptoms. Typical incubation periods are one to three days for the common cold and influenza, two to five days for diphtheria and gonorrhoea, one to two weeks for measles and whooping cough, two to three weeks for chicken pox, mumps and German measles (rubella), and one and three months for hepatitis A and B respectively.

Typical features of diseases caused by particular bacteria and viruses are shown in tables 3.1 and 3.2 (pages 80 and 82). Occasionally the clinical effects are characteristic of one micro-organism (e.g. measles). More often a particular clinical picture can be caused by one of a number of different organisms. We shall briefly consider two conditions in this latter category, namely sore throats and pneumonia.

Sore throats

Sore throats are among the commonest conditions seen in general practice, especially in the winter. Most are caused by viruses and most resolve completely in a few days without any special treatment. The inflammation may involve the pharynx (the part of the alimentary canal just beyond the mouth) or the tonsils (two small lumps of lymphoid tissue, one on each side of the throat at the upper end of the pharynx). Some bacteria cause sore throats requiring medical attention. In diphtheria the inflammatory reaction is sometimes so severe that it obstructs the airway. Streptococcus pyogenes is a common cause of acute tonsillitis; diagnosis is important in view of potentially serious reactions in some patients (e.g. rheumatic fever, nephritis). Sore throat is a symptom, not necessarily the main one, in many diseases. When recurrent it may be a sign of increased susceptibility to infection. Protracted, recurrent or severe sore throat deserves medical attention, if only to exclude the more serious causes.

Pneumonia

Bacteria, viruses and other organisms can cause pneumonia. Bacterial infections are the commonest. In one kind of pneumonia the inflammatory process starts in the alveoli and works upwards, so that a discrete region of lung becomes densely affected. This is **lobar pneumonia**, typically due to **Streptococcus pneumoniae**. In another kind, **bronchopneumonia**, the organisms spread down the bronchial tree causing a patchy but widespread infection involving both lungs. It tends to occur when there is some predisposing condition, such as bronchitis, lung damage or a debilitating illness. Pneumonia impairs gas-exchange in the lung and may cause hypoxia (oxygen deficiency). Typical symptoms of pneumonia are fever, cough and breathlessness. In lobar pneumonia there is often a characteristic sharp chest pain on inspiration or coughing. It is due to inflammation of the pleura, the membrane covering the lung (a condition called **pleurisy**). Untreated, the mortality of acute pneumonia can be high, especially when there is another underlying lung disorder. With the correct antibiotic treatment there is usually rapid and complete recovery. Occasionally pneumonia results in permanent lung damage.

Other symptoms of infection

Fever (**pyrexia**) is an abnormally high body temperature. It is a general accompaniment of inflammation, especially that due to infection. Its purpose, if any, is unknown. The normal internal body temperature is $37^{\circ}C$. Substances released by the inflammatory process affect the temperature regulation centre in the brain, which sets its thermostat at a higher level. In some infections the temperature swings up and down quite markedly, sometimes characteristically. When the temperature is too high the blood vessels in the skin dilate to give off heat and the patient sweats and feels hot. When the temperature reaches the lower level the body reacts by conserving and producing heat. The skin vessels close down, causing chilliness, and the muscles start to shiver (**rigor**). A feeling of unease (**malaise**), loss of appetite and headache often accompany fever.

Severe bacterial infections occasionally produce a dangerous form of shock (inadequate blood flow in vital tissues and organs).

HIV infection

The **human immunodeficiency virus** (**HIV**) causes the **acquired immunodeficiency syndrome** (**AIDS**), a condition in which the body loses its ability to resist infection. AIDS is a new human disease. It was first recognised in a few previously healthy homosexual men in the US in 1981. The disease was already prevalent in Africa, which still has the biggest burden of HIV infection. In North America and Europe the disease initially spread mainly through male homosexual and intravenous drug abuse practices. Heterosexual transmission is now also of major concern in these continents, and it appears always to have been the predominant form of transmission in Sub-Saharan Africa where men and women are equally affected.

HIV attacks a particular type of lymphocyte known as the **CD4+ helper T-lymphocyte** (hereafter called the **CD4 cell**). This cell has a pivotal role in the regulation of the immune system. Its depletion in AIDS leaves the patient particularly susceptible to infections by viruses, fungi, protozoa and some bacteria. HIV also attacks the nervous system. HIV is not particularly infectious and the organism is fragile. The infection is not contracted through normal non-sexual social contact nor by being in proximity to someone with AIDS. It is spread through unprotected anal and vaginal intercourse, and by injection of infected blood and blood products.

The first definite indication of infection is the detection in the serum of antibodies to HIV (antibody positive). This sero-conversion occurs three weeks to three months after exposure to the infection; in a few people this is accompanied by a febrile illness with symptoms similar to some other virus infections. In most it goes unnoticed. The incubation period for HIV ranges from one to more than ten years. Because of the long course of the disease and the short time that has been available for its study, there is some uncertainty about how many HIV infected people will not develop AIDS. For homosexual and bisexual men there is evidence that half may remain free of AIDS ten years after infection.

There are strict diagnostic criteria for the different clinical presentations of HIV infection; the clinical course (the development of symptoms) varies considerably. AIDS is the label given to the final stage of HIV infection in which particular micro-organisms and tumours take the opportunity to invade the severely immune-compromised host. At this stage the CD4 cell count is usually below 200 cells per cubic millimetre of blood; the normal reference range is 800-1200. The commonest opportunistic infection is **Pneumocystis carinii pneumonia** (PCP), which is a major cause of death in AIDS. Pneumocystis carinii is usually classified as a protozoan. The pneumonia often first presents as a chronic cough. A tumour known as **Kaposi's sarcoma** is also a typical feature, particularly in homosexual or bisexual men with AIDS. It may appear as red or purple patches on the head, neck, trunk or limbs, and it may affect the respiratory or digestive tracts. AIDS is invariably fatal; most patients die within two years of developing the full-blown disease. Anti-infective drug therapy has extended and improved life for many patients with AIDS, but there is as yet no cure available.

– Abnormal immune reactions - allergy –

Introduction

The immune response is protective and normally benefits the patient. When a foreign antigen enters the body the immune system produces antibodies to it. The antibody locks onto and forms a complex with specific, recognised, parts of the molecular structure of the antigen. This may neutralise the toxic effect of the antigen or prepare it for further attack by other immune system devices. Sometimes the immune-system directs T-lymphocytes against the antigen.

Antigens are usually proteins. The body contains thousands of different proteins and the walls of its cells contain many potential antigens. Normally, the immune system only reacts against foreign antigens. At an early stage it learns to distinguish self from non-self.

Occasionally, however, the immune system responds abnormally and actually causes or augments disease. It may over-react to external foreign proteins, as in hay fever and some forms of asthma and eczema, or direct its activities against the body's own tissues (**auto-immune disease**), as in rheumatic fever, rheumatoid arthritis and some types of diabetes mellitus and thyroid gland disease. The abnormal immune response may occur very soon after exposure to the antigen or after a delay of one or more days (delayed-type hypersensitivity).

In some forms of nephritis the presence of **immune-complexes** consisting of a conglomeration of antibody and antigen molecules appears to trigger the inflammatory response in the kidneys. In many cases the nephritis occurs one to three weeks after a streptococcal sore throat.

The term **allergy** usually refers to an abnormal immune response in which there is an increased sensitivity to an external substance.

The immediate hypersensitivity response

The commonest type of abnormal immune reaction involves a class of antibody known as **IgE**. Individuals sensitive to particular substances produce an excess of the corresponding IgE antibodies. IgE sits on the surface of special cells (**mast cells**) present in the tissues. When the antigen interacts with IgE the mast cell releases chemicals which cause an acute inflammatory response. One of the substances released is **histamine** which causes some of the earliest features of inflammation, such as dilation of small blood vessels and an increase in their permeability, which lead to local redness and oedema. Histamine also causes itching. Because the antibodies are already present and the mast cells have a stock of chemicals ready for release, this type of immune reaction often starts within minutes of exposure; it is sometimes called **immediate hypersensitivity**. This is the archetypal allergic reaction. It causes hay fever, bad reactions to bee stings, hives (an itchy skin rash with weals) and some forms of asthma and eczema.

Hay fever is a common name for **seasonal allergic rhinitis** which is an allergy to antigenic pollens from grasses, flowers, weeds or trees. The commonest cause in the UK is grass pollen; in North America it is ragweed. The condition is very common and occurs in the spring and summer. Mast cells in the membranes lining the nasal passages react to antigens reaching them from the air. The acute inflammation that follows causes a stuffy and profusely runny nose, and much sneezing. Fever is unusual.

A few people are extremely allergic to a particular substance which if taken into the body, by injection or sometimes by mouth, can cause a severe widespread immediate hypersensitivity reaction (**systemic anaphylaxis**). The condition is rare but can be life-threatening.

Delayed-type hypersensitivity

T-lymphocytes play a major role in this type of response. **Delayed-type hypersensitivity** (**DTH**) causes the chronic inflammation seen in chronic infections such as tuberculosis and syphilis. The immune system attempts to contain the infection but the accompanying inflammatory reaction is also destructive to surrounding healthy tissue.

DTH is the mechanism behind **allergic contact dermatitis**, a skin rash caused by contact with particular substances of small molecular size. Culprits include nickel (present in some jewellery and garment clips), some chemicals in cement, hair dyes, rubber, cosmetics, perfumes and sticking plasters, some drugs used on the skin, and substances in plants such as primula and poison ivy. The offending substance combines with protein in the skin to form a new antigen (known as a **hapten**) which is then able to stimulate an immune response. It may take some time, and possibly several exposures, for people to become fully sensitised. Once a person is sensitised the rash is usually obvious within two days of exposure to the substance.

Bronchial asthma

Bronchial asthma is a common disease characterised by recurrent episodes of breathlessness due to widespread narrowing of the bronchial air passages in the lungs. Often the disease starts in childhood or early adult life, and there may be a family history of hay fever or eczema. In such cases asthma is usually due to the inhalation of antigens which activate

IgE-bearing mast cells in the lungs and cause an immediate hypersensitivity response. Other mechanisms operate too, but they are less well defined. Substances released during the inflammatory reaction stimulate spasm of the muscles in the bronchial wall and the formation of mucus in the small airways; both events cause airways obstruction.

Allergens (antigens) known to precipitate attacks of asthma include pollens, fungi, animal dander (hair and feather particles) and house dust. Important allergens in house dust come from the house-dust mite, a minute creature which lives in bedding and likes human skin scales and secretions. Patients are usually sensitive to more than one allergen. Smoke, cold air and exercise can also trigger attacks. Some asthmatics are not allergic to external antigens and have a different form of the disease.

Asthma attacks may last for hours or days. Many patients are relatively symptom-free between attacks, some have a more chronic form. Typical clinical features are a feeling of tightness in the chest, shortness of breath and wheezing. So-called **severe acute asthma** is life-threatening and the patient's condition can deteriorate rapidly. Very poor ventilation in the alveoli results in dangerous hypoxaemia (lack of oxygen – see chapter two, page 36). Severe acute asthma is a medical emergency requiring urgent treatment. Fortunately, most episodes of asthma resolve uneventfully, especially with the help of modern medicines. Some patients require continuous maintenance therapy to keep well. Childhood asthma occasionally disappears completely.

Rheumatic fever and rheumatic heart disease

Rheumatism is a vague term commonly used to describe aches and pains in joints, muscles and connective tissues. There are many causes. Rheumatic fever, rheumatic heart disease and rheumatoid arthritis are names given to particular clinical entities. Abnormal immune responses occur in these disorders. Rheumatoid arthritis is more conveniently considered in a later section, on page 99.

In rheumatic fever there is a sterile inflammation of the joints (**arthritis**), heart (**carditis**), skin and occasionally the brain.

It starts two to four weeks after a sore throat caused by specific strains of Streptococcus pyogenes. There are no organisms in the affected tissues. The antibodies produced against the Streptococcus also cross-react with certain healthy tissues, including the myocardium and heart valves. Only a small proportion of people are prone to rheumatic fever after streptococcal sore throats; there is an individual variation in susceptibility.

Rheumatic fever occurs mainly in children and young adults. Clinical features include fever, pain and tenderness in one or more joints and sometimes a skin rash. Carditis varies in severity and may be absent. When severe it can cause heart failure. A few patients develop **chorea**, a brain disorder characterised by involuntary jerky flailing movements of the limbs (St Vitus's dance). Rheumatic fever may last for many weeks and require a prolonged period of bed rest. Most patients recover completely.

An important long-term complication in some is the persistence of a chronic inflammatory process in the heart valves, despite apparent recovery from rheumatic fever. This is chronic rheumatic heart disease and it can lead to significant valve damage. The interval between rheumatic fever and the appearance of symptoms from valvular heart disease may be five to thirty years. The process particularly affects the mitral valve, which becomes narrowed (**mitral stenosis**) or leaky, allowing backflow (variously called **mitral incompetence**, **regurgitation** or **reflux**). Valve damage may progress to the point where it eventually causes clinical illness, such as breathlessness and heart failure. Surgical treatment is usually possible and successful.

Food allergy

Many substances taken by mouth are potential antigens but the body is normally able to tolerate them without producing dangerous immune responses. Occasionally, certain foods, food additives and contaminants do cause hypersensitivity reactions in susceptible individuals. These may take the form of gastro-intestinal symptoms (e.g. vomiting, diarrhoea), hives, asthma or, rarely, even systemic anaphylaxis (this may present as bronchospasm and shock). Food allergies can be very specific but often the agent responsible is not identified. Foods that have been associated with hypersensitivity reactions include eggs, fish, shellfish, milk, nuts, chocolate and some fruits.

In a few susceptible individuals a protein called **gluten**, which is present in wheat and some other cereals, causes a delayed-type hypersensitivity response in the lining of the small bowel. In young children this gives rise to **coeliac disease**, in which impaired food absorption retards physical development. Gluten hypersensitivity in adults causes diarrhoea.

Short monographs on particular diseases

The following diseases are commonly seen in general practice and hospital. They will help further to consolidate your knowledge and understanding of some aspects of medicine.

Arthritis

The term arthritis is commonly applied to a number of disorders of the joints. The commonest, **osteoarthritis**, is not primarily an inflammatory disease. Infection or chemical deposits in a joint (as in the metabolic disease **gout**) can cause an inflammatory arthritis. Rheumatic fever and rheumatoid arthritis are examples of abnormal immune responses that cause joint inflammation.

A joint that allows significant movement is a **synovial joint**; the basic features are shown in figure 3.5. The two bones in the joint do not glide directly over each other. Their ends are protected by thin but tough, springy layers of gristle called the **articular cartilages**. The smooth free surfaces of the cartilages (the **articular surfaces**) glide over each other assisted by a special lubricant, the **synovial fluid**. The weight-bearing joints such as the hip, knee and ankle must withstand tremendous stresses over many years. The special properties of cartilage and synovial fluid help protect the apposing (touching) bone ends from damage. The joint is surrounded and protected

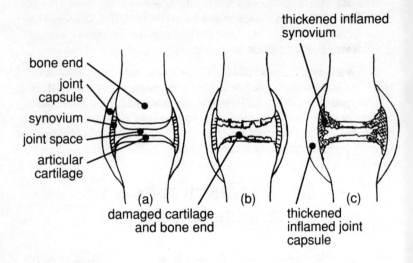

Figure 3.5 The synovial joint and arthritis
(a) Normal
(b) Osteoarthritis
(c) Rheumatoid arthritis

by the joint capsule, the outer layer of which is tough and fibrous. Lining the inside of the joint capsule but not extending over the articular surfaces is the **synovium**, a cellular membrane which produces the special lubricating polymer of the synovial fluid.

Osteoarthritis

Osteoarthritis is a degeneration of the articular surfaces, initially eroding the cartilage and later the bone ends. It particularly affects the weight-bearing joints. Abnormal stresses and strains and the associated wear and tear on the joint are probably important factors in its progression, although the precise initiating cause is often unknown. Other joint and bone disorders, including trauma, predispose to the condition. Most old people have some degree of osteoarthritis, although in many it is mild and may not always produce symptoms. To some extent it may be regarded as part of the aging process. However, osteoarthritis can be severe and disabling, and it can affect younger people. Inflammation does occur but it is generally secondary to joint damage rather than the cause of it.

Rheumatoid arthritis

Rheumatoid arthritis is a chronic inflammatory disease which affects several joints and sometimes involves other tissues and organs. It affects about one per cent of the population, women more than men, and usually starts in the third to fifth decades. The inflammatory reaction starts in the synovium, which becomes thickened and infiltrated with T-lymphocytes. As the disease progresses the inflamed tissue encroaches onto and then damages the articular surfaces (see figure 3.5). What initiates the disease is not known, but once started the chronic inflammatory process seems to be self-perpetuating. Some individuals are more genetically predisposed to rheumatoid arthritis than others.

Typically, rheumatoid arthritis starts gradually in the small joints of the hands and feet, and then spreads to the wrists, elbows and other joints. The hip is often spared. The arthritis is similar on both sides. The disease is prone to repeated attacks and remissions. Each attack produces further structural damage and loss of function. The affected joints are swollen, warm and painful, and stiff first thing in the morning. Some patients have many relapses over many years leading to a variable degree of disability. A few are severely crippled. Some have a limited disease from which they recover completely. Powerful drugs can dampen the inflammatory response and provide considerable relief, but sometimes they may cause additional problems.

Chronic bronchitis

The clinical hallmark of chronic bronchitis is a cough with the production of phlegm (sputum) from the lungs on most days for a period of at least three months each year for more than two consecutive years. The disease usually occurs in middle age or later and progresses over several years. It is a major cause of disability and death in the UK.

Tobacco smoke and many atmospheric pollutants irritate the bronchial epithelium. Persistent irritation eventually leads to the permanent changes of chronic bronchitis in which there is an increased number of mucus-producing cells in the bronchial tree. Smoking, pollution, upper respiratory tract infections, and cold and damp conditions encourage the production of excessive amounts of mucus-containing (mucoid) sputum. Poor clearance of mucus encourages the growth of bacteria in the lower respiratory tract. People with chronic bronchitis are prone to recurrent lung infections with purulent sputum, especially during the winter.

Smoking and infection stimulate phagocytes in the lung to release enzymes which incidentally damage the structure of the air-exchange units. This may eventually lead to **emphysema**, a permanent enlargement of the air spaces at the ends of the bronchial tree, a condition that impairs gas-exchange. Some patients have an increased genetic predisposition to emphysema. The lung damage in severe chronic bronchitis sometimes causes hypoxaemia and respiratory failure (see chapter two, page 36). Infection and obstruction of the airways by mucus may cause a sudden and dangerous deterioration in such cases.

Oxygen therapy is often necessary for patients with chronic bronchitis and respiratory failure, but it must be carefully controlled. In these patients too much oxygen can actually depress the drive to breathe. In some patients with respiratory failure the carbon dioxide levels in the blood are abnormally high, which causes additional problems. Anything which depresses breathing in these circumstances can induce dangerously high carbon dioxide levels. Narcotic and sedative drugs also depress respiration and are dangerous for these patients.

The course of the disease and the extent of emphysema varies considerably from patient to patient. In some there is little inconvenience apart from the nuisance of the cough. In others the disease causes severe breathlessness and disability and takes a downhill course over relatively few years.

Diabetes mellitus

Diabetes mellitus is characterised by an abnormally high concentration of glucose in the blood (**hyperglycaemia**). It affects more than two per cent of the population.

The disease is caused by a lack of insulin or by a lack of response to insulin. The action of this hormone on glucose metabolism was described in chapter two, page 49. Insulin deficiency impairs glucose uptake by the cells and results in abnormally high blood glucose levels in the fasting state and after a meal. In most people the renal tubules reabsorb glucose completely at all normal blood glucose levels, so that none appears in the urine. There is a limit to the kidney's ability. In diabetes the levels are too high and glucose spills into the urine, a simple screening test for the disease. A high urine glucose concentration exerts an osmotic effect which retains more water than usual in the renal tubule. Therefore the patient passes large amounts of urine, feels thirsty and drinks a lot to keep up with the water loss. Untreated, severe hyperglycaemia can lead to serious dehydration, and ultimately coma and death.

There are two types of diabetes mellitus; **type 1** which occurs in young people, almost always before 40 years, and requires insulin injections; and **type 2** which is commoner, occurs in those over 40 years and which does not usually require treatment with insulin. Type 1 is an auto-immune disease in which the body produces antibodies to the B cells of the pancreas. The ensuing inflammatory response gradually destroys the insulin-producing cells. Clinical symptoms appear when the production of insulin is inadequate to meet needs; this occurs after about 80 to 90 per cent of the cells have been destroyed. Normally plasma insulin levels increase in response to a rise in plasma glucose, after a meal for instance. In type 1 diabetes plasma insulin is low or absent. What initiates the disease is not known. There appears to be a genetic predisposition in some but this is not a matter of simple single gene inheritance and environmental factors, such as viral infections, may be important too.

There is no abnormal immune reaction to B cells in type 2 diabetes. Plasma insulin may be normal or even increased but the response of the body's cells to insulin is diminished, and the net effect is one of insulin deficiency. The genetic influence is stronger than, but different to, that in type 1. Both genetic and environmental factors are important and dietary factors may also play a role in its development. The majority of type 2 diabetics are obese, but the majority of obese people are not diabetic. The progression of type 2 (or late-onset) diabetes is generally much slower and less dramatic but the end result can be as serious and the long-term medical complications of the disease are similar in both types. Weight control and reduction of the carbohydrate content in the diet, most of which converts to glucose, often reduces plasma glucose to acceptable levels in late-onset (type 2) diabetes. Special medicines which can be taken by mouth are sometimes given in addition to the diet to squeeze more insulin from the pancreatic islet B cells. Occasionally these measures fail and insulin injections are necessary as in type 1 diabetes.

Typical clinical features of untreated diabetes mellitus are the passing of large volumes of urine (**polyuria**), thirst and recurrent infections, such as thrush in the genital regions and abscesses. Occasionally patients with severe diabetes, usually type 1, present for the first time in a state of near, or actual, coma.

Coma or near coma is a grave complication of diabetes. Good management should prevent it. One type of coma arises when inadequate (or no) treatment leads to very high blood glucose levels and severe dehydration. In type 1 diabetes there may also be a serious increase in hydrogen-ion formation, which may cause gasping respirations. In fact there are many metabolic changes and they present special therapeutic challenges, even for experienced doctors. The other type of coma is caused by an overdose of insulin which produces a low blood glucose level (**hypoglycaemia**). Severe hypoglycaemia can damage the brain permanently within minutes.

Both types of diabetes mellitus are prone to serious long-term complications. Atherosclerosis occurs earlier and is more severe than in non-diabetics, leading to a higher mortality from cardiovascular and cerebrovascular disease. Another process damages the small blood vessels of the retina (in the eyes) and the kidneys, which may eventually cause blindness and renal failure respectively. Diabetes may affect the peripheral nerves or the autonomic nervous system, giving rise to a host of different ill effects. In some patients the vascular and neurological abnormalities and the high glucose levels in the tissues encourage the development of infected ulcers and gangrene, especially in the toes and feet.

Although there is no cure as yet for diabetes mellitus, many patients can live a long and relatively trouble-free life on modern treatment. Good management of diabetes aims to keep blood glucose as close as possible to normal levels without the risk of hypoglycaemia. An increasing body of evidence indicates that strict control over a long period reduces the incidence of serious long-term complications.

Peptic ulcer

A **peptic ulcer** is an open sore in the lining of the digestive tract in an area exposed to the effects of acid gastric juice. It may develop in the stomach (**gastric ulcer**) or in the first part of the duodenum just beyond the outlet of the stomach (**duodenal ulcer**). Duodenal ulcers are commoner, affect men more than women and occur mainly in the third and fourth decades. Gastric ulcers tend to occur in the fourth and fifth decades. Probably at least one in twenty people develop a peptic ulcer at some time in their life.

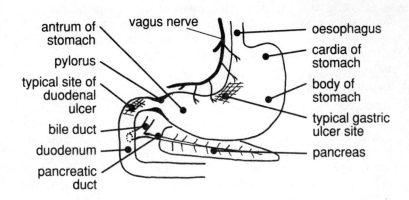

Figure 3.6 The stomach and duodenum

The stomach is divided anatomically into the **fundus** (the upper part farthest away from the outlet), the body and the **antrum**, which passes to the gateway (**pylorus**) controlling the entry of partially digested food into the duodenum (see figure 3.6). The acid gastric juice arises from special epithelial cells (**parietal cells**) in the fundus and body of the stomach. The thought, sight, smell or taste of food causes nervous stimulation of gastric acid production. The **vagus nerves** carry the signals to the stomach. The presence of food protein in the stomach stimulates cells in the antrum to release the hormone **gastrin**, which in turn stimulates the formation of more gastric juice. Locally produced histamine also plays an important role in acid production by stimulating receptors on the parietal cells. Other cells protect the lining of the stomach from digestion by producing an **antacid** (bicarbonate) and a layer of mucus.

Increased acid production is a factor in the development of some duodenal ulcers, and the presence of acid gastric juice retards the healing of established peptic ulcers. Impaired protection of the epithelial surface is probably an important factor in ulcer development. There is now compelling evidence that the main underlying cause of many peptic ulcers is a chronic inflammation of the antrum caused by the bacillus **Helicobacter pylori** which, unlike most micro-organisms, can live in the hostile environment of the stomach. Smoking and stress may also contribute to peptic ulceration, and there is also a familial tendency. Aspirin can cause acute inflammation and erosions in the lining of the stomach.

The main symptom is upper abdominal pain or discomfort. There may be nausea or vomiting. Occasionally, erosion of a blood vessel in the floor of the ulcer produces a sudden large haemorrhage, causing the patient to vomit blood (**haematemesis**) and/or to pass black tarry stools (**melaena**). Chronic seepage of blood may lead to anaemia. Another possible complication is perforation through the wall of the stomach or duodenum, allowing gastric material to enter the abdominal cavity and cause a severe reaction (e.g. peritonitis). Although peptic ulceration can be very distressing and debilitating it is now an uncommon cause of death. Very occasionally malignant change may occur in a gastric ulcer, or a gastric carcinoma may masquerade as an ulcer. Persistent gastric ulcers therefore require extra investigation.

A reduction in gastric acid promotes the healing of peptic ulcers. Substances that neutralise the acid in the stomach (antacids) can be used but they are less effective and have more side effects than the preferred treatment with modern drugs that suppress the production of hydrogen ions by the parietal cells (see chapter nine, page 204). However, such treatment must often be continued for long periods to prevent recurrence of the ulcer. The success of modern drug treatment has dramatically reduced the need for surgical treatment although surgery is sometimes necessary, especially when there are serious complications. Traditional surgical procedures include cutting the vagus nerves to the stomach to reduce excessive acid formation in some patients with duodenal ulcer and removing the ulcer together with the gastrin-secreting region of the stomach in some patients with gastric ulcer. Antibacterial treatment of Helicobacter pylori infection offers hope of a more permanent medical cure for peptic ulcer, at least in some patients. Trials are in progress.

4
GENETIC DISORDERS

Revision of the sections on cells, genes, proteins and reproduction in chapter two may be advantageous to the reader at this point.

—— Types of genetic disorder ——

Genetic diseases arise from defects in particular genes, either single or multiple, or from chromosome abnormalities. Although most are uncommon, together they form an important and formidable challenge to modern medicine. They are a major cause of suffering and death in childhood.

Chromosomal disorders are caused by an abnormal number of whole chromosomes in the cell or abnormal structural rearrangements of large chunks. Such cellular abnormalities can usually be seen with the microscope using special techniques. These faults arise during the formation of the ovum or sperm; the causes are poorly understood. About 0.5 per cent of live-born babies have a chromosome abnormality. One of the commonest and best known is **Down's syndrome** (see page 114).

So far, about 5,000 different clinical entities due to single gene abnormalities have been recorded. The precise nature of the defect in many of these is still unknown, but in some the genetic abnormalities and the mechanisms by which they cause disease have been worked out in great detail. Most of the single gene disorders are rare but as a group they affect about 1 per cent of live-born babies in the UK.

We have already seen how changes in DNA during life can lead to cancer. Such changes in a person's non-reproductive cells are not passed on to their children. However, genetic defects in the germ cells responsible for reproduction may be passed on to future generations and appear in all the cells of the affected offspring. This is how the inheritable genetic disorders arise. The single-gene defect has a relatively simple mode of inheritance.

Some of our characteristics, such as weight and build, depend on the activities of many genes and the effects of non-genetic factors such as diet and physical activity. Multiple genes probably influence the clinical expression of some disorders that appear in later life and show familial trends, such as hypertension, atherosclerosis, diabetes, asthma and schizophrenia, and also some of the congenital abnormalities (present at birth) such as cleft lip (harelip) and cleft palate. Inheritance is less clear cut in these than in the single-gene disorders. Environmental factors sometimes modify the course and severity of genetically-determined diseases.

The basis of inheritable genetic disorders

A gene is represented in a specific segment of DNA in a chromosome. It determines the structure and therefore the function of a particular protein chain. A small change in DNA structure can adversely affect protein manufacture. This may result in the production of too little protein, or in the production of a variant or faulty protein. DNA structure can be affected in a number of ways. In many instances there is a change in just one of the base units (A,T,G or C; see chapter two, page 16). A new change in DNA structure is a **mutation**. Once present in the germ cell the modification can be transferred to future generations. Such mutations occur spontaneously in the population, some more frequently than others.

A change in a DNA base unit may cause substitution of the wrong amino acid at the corresponding point in the protein chain. This may or may not significantly alter the ability of the protein to function properly. Some parts of the protein molecule are more important determinants of its function and stability than others. Whether or not such a change in function at the molecular level will cause disease depends on other factors too. Thus, a single-gene defect may or may not cause disease, and when it does the severity of the disease can vary considerably.

Sex-chromosomes and autosomes

The nucleus of a germ cell contains 23 chromosomes. Only one of these chromosomes determines sexual characteristics: it is either an X-chromosome, which endows female properties, or a Y-chromosome, which confers maleness. An ovum contains only an X-chromosome whereas a sperm may carry either an X- or a Y- chromosome. After conception, the zygote (first cell of a new being) will contain 46 chromosomes, two of which are sex-chromosomes. There is an approximately equal chance that the X-carrying ovum will unite with an X- or a Y-carrying sperm, to give either an XX or an XY combination in the zygote, and therefore the cells arising from it. People with XX combinations in their cells are female and those with XY are male. About 0.2 per cent of the population have abnormal numbers of sex chromosomes in their cells.

In a normal female cell only one of the two X-chromosomes is active. The other is inactive and appears as a discrete mass near the nuclear membrane. This distinct nuclear body is known as **sex-chromatin** and is easily seen in accessible cells (e.g. from a gentle scraping of the inside lining of the cheek) using simple microscopic techniques. The inactivation of one or other of the X-chromosomes in female cells affects those of maternal and paternal origin approximately equally. Normal male cells have only one X-chromosome, which is fully active, and therefore no sex-chromatin. This provides a simple test for genetic sex status. The expression of sexual characteristics in men and women depends on other factors too.

The other chromosomes are known as **autosomes**. Ordinary cells contain two matching sets of 22 autosomes, one set from each parent. Each matching pair of chromosomes contains a set of matching genes. Each matching pair of genes is responsible for the production of a protein chain with a specific function, but either one of the pair can produce it.

When a disease is caused by an abnormal gene on the X-chromosome it is said to be **X-linked** or **sex-linked**. (The X-chromosome contains many genes that have functions other than sex determination.) Diseases arising from abnormal genes on the autosomes are said to be **autosomal**.

Dominant and recessive single gene disorders

Sometimes only one gene in a matching pair needs to be abnormal to produce disease; the remaining normal gene is unable to compensate. Such diseases and their mode of inheritance are said to be **dominant**. Other genetic diseases do not reveal themselves unless both genes are affected; they are said to be **recessive**. People who have one normal gene and one defective gene for a recessive genetic disorder do not usually manifest the disease, but they are **carriers** of the affected gene and they can pass it to their offspring. There are many **autosomal dominant** and **autosomal recessive** disorders.

There are fewer X-linked diseases and they are mostly recessive. Although X-linked recessive disorders do not usually affect the female carrier, they always affect those males who inherit the affected gene because they have only one X-chromosome and therefore no back-up healthy gene to compensate for the defect. The female carrier can pass either her healthy or defective X-linked gene to her offspring. If she mates with an unaffected male there is a one in two chance that any son will be affected and a one in two chance that any daughter will be a carrier. If an affected male mates with a completely normal female then none of their male children will get the disease but all of their daughters will be carriers. This is because paternal X-chromosomes go to daughters, not sons.

Haemophilia

Haemophilia is a well known X-linked recessive disease in which affected males suffer from a marked tendency to bleed, particularly into the joints and muscles. In the commonest form the gene involved normally codes for a plasma protein called **factor VIII** which is an important part of the normal blood clotting system. The factor is markedly deficient in the plasma of severely affected males and partially deficient in carrier females, who have about half the normal complement of normal X-linked factor VIII genes (because of the random inactivation of either the paternal or maternal X-chromosome – see the previous section).

Haemophilia illustrates an important point. Although female carriers of the gene do not usually suffer from the disease, which is therefore clinically recessive, they do have abnormally low plasma factor VIII levels. So in terms of biochemical expression the disease is not strictly recessive, and in a few cases the biochemical abnormality in the carrier may be sufficient to cause some clinical effect. In some autosomal and sex-linked genetic disorders the carriers of one abnormal gene suffer from a less severe form of the disease. Thus, the terms dominant and recessive are relative and there is a grey area between them.

Autosomal inheritance

Autosomal inheritance affects males and females similarly. A severe autosomal dominant disorder is likely to become rapidly extinct because there are no disease-free carriers to pass on the genes and affected patients are less likely to breed. Thus, dominant genetic diseases tend to be less severe, but there are exceptions. In **Huntington's disease** the onset of symptoms usually starts in middle age, so patients may already have had children. The disease affects the brain and progresses relentlessly causing mental deterioration and chorea (involuntary jerky movements) and death within about 15 years of onset.

A person with an autosomal dominant disease generally has only one affected gene per cell; the corresponding gene on the matching chromosome is normal. If they mate with a genetically normal partner any child conceived has a one in two chance of inheriting the disease.

In some autosomal dominant conditions clinical expression of the abnormal gene may be quite variable between affected individuals, even within the same family. In such cases other genes and environmental factors may modify the effect of the abnormal gene.

An autosomal dominant disease can often be traced through several generations. The same is not true of autosomal recessive diseases which often arise unexpectedly with no previous family history. In most autosomal recessive disorders the carriers, who possess one affected gene, are clinically completely normal. These diseases most often appear for the first time in a family when two unsuspecting carriers mate. Many autosomal recessive diseases are rare; when this is the case the likelihood of two carriers mating is small. Furthermore, there is only a one in four chance that any child from two carrier parents will be clinically affected.

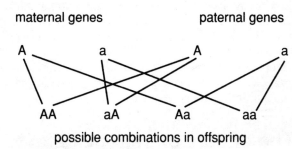

maternal genes   paternal genes

possible combinations in offspring

AA = genetically and clinically normal
Aa, aA = carrier, like parents
aa = clinically affected

where A = normal gene
   a = recessive affected gene

Figure 4.1 Autosomal recessive inheritance

Figure 4.1 illustrates the possible genetic combinations that can occur when two carriers of an autosomal recessive disease produce offspring. For any pregnancy there is a 25 per cent chance that the child will inherit the abnormal gene from both parents and therefore get the disease. There is a 50 per cent chance that the child will receive just one abnormal gene per cell and so be a symptomless carrier like the parents. There is also a 25 per cent chance that the child will be clinically and genetically completely normal with respect to that disease by inheriting only the healthy genes from each parent. There is an element of chance in the inheritance of genes and the figures described merely represent a statistical probability. Occasionally carrier parents may be unfortunate enough to have two or more affected children in a row, whereas others may only have clinically normal offspring and will never be aware of the presence of abnormal genes.

If the occurrence of symptomless carriers for a particular autosomal recessive disease is say one in every fifty people, then the chance of two carriers becoming nuptial partners is one in every two and a half thousand such relationships (i.e. 50^2). As stated above, the chance of any resultant pregnancy being affected by the disease is one in four. This means that the frequency of the disease in the population at large would be only one in ten thousand births. Many autosomal recessive disorders are rarer than this. Cystic fibrosis affects approximately one in every two thousand live births (in Caucasians); the reader may wish to confirm that the frequency of carriers in the population is therefore about one in twenty-two.

—— The effects of genetic defects ——

Genetic disorders may be obvious at birth or they may not become apparent until later in infancy, childhood or even adulthood. Whatever the age of onset the course and severity of the diseases can vary tremendously. Some are mild and compatible with a normal life span, some are rapidly fatal in childhood, others pursue a relentless and debilitating course over many years. Genetic abnormalities are very common in the products of spontaneous (natural) abortions in which the mother's body rejects the embryo soon after conception; presumably many are incompatible with life.

Many chromosome defects cause internal and external physical abnormalities, and sometimes a characteristic appearance. Learning disability (mental retardation) is common.

In a single-gene disease the genetic defect usually affects the function of a particular protein. The protein may be part of the fabric of a cell or tissue, or have a highly specific activity as a hormone, enzyme, or chemical receptor or transporter. The inherited disorders of haemoglobin illustrate different ways in which protein manufacture may be affected (these are the commonest single-gene diseases worldwide). In one type (**thalassaemia**) there is inadequate production of globin chains, whereas in another (**sickle-cell disease**) a globin of abnormal structure is produced (see page 115).

When an enzyme is affected there may be a serious metabolic disturbance. An enzyme facilitates and speeds up a particular chemical reaction; it is a specific biological catalyst. There are thousands of different chemical reactions in the body, and so there are thousands of specific enzymes. A deficiency in the activity of an enzyme may impair conversion of one chemical (say A) into another (say B). This may lead to an excess and sometimes an accumulation of A and a deficiency of B. The clinical effect of this depends on the toxicity of A (and its by-products) and whether B is essential and cannot be obtained in the required amount by other means. For example, in the autosomal recessive disease **phenylketonuria** there is a deficiency of the liver enzyme responsible for the conversion of the amino acid **phenylalanine** into another amino acid, **tyrosine**. When the affected infant takes normal protein in its diet (e.g. from milk) there is an abnormal increase in the plasma phenylalanine concentration which, uncorrected, can retard normal mental development.

Enzymes are usually present in excess of requirements. So carriers of one defective gene for an enzyme are often clinically normal because the corresponding gene on the paired chromosome makes sufficient normal enzyme to cope, even though there may be only half the usual amount present. For this reason most enzyme deficiency diseases are recessive.

Single-gene disorders are responsible for a vast array of clinical conditions. They may affect the form or function of various parts of the body and some cause learning disability (mental retardation). Some single-gene diseases have characteristic clinical features. However, sometimes defects in quite distinct genes produce similar clinical pictures, and different defects in a particular gene may produce different clinical effects with considerable variation in severity.

Down's syndrome

Down's syndrome is a chromosome abnormality affecting about one in seven hundred live births overall, but the incidence increases with maternal age and it affects up to one per cent of births in mothers over 40 years.

The different autosomes are identified by numbers, 1 to 22. Normal individuals have a pair of each in every cell (apart from germ cells, which have just one set). People with Down's syndrome have a chromosome 21 abnormality, usually three are present instead of the pair (**21-trisomy**).

Typically, the face looks flat, the eyes are slanted and the tongue protrudes through an open mouth. There are other structural anomalies, often a heart defect, and a learning disability (mental retardation). The severity of the condition varies. People with Down's syndrome often have a pleasant happy personality. Death sometimes occurs in early childhood. Many survive to adulthood but they tend to age prematurely and are prone to dementia (see chapter five, page 129).

Sickle-cell anaemia

This autosomal recessive disease of the red blood cells particularly affects Black people of African origin. Apparently the carrier status confers some genetic advantage by providing a degree of protection against a dangerous form of malaria. The frequency of carriers, who have one affected gene per cell is as high as one in every three to four people in some parts of equatorial Africa, and is about one in ten in Black Americans. Unfortunately, inheritance of two sickle-cell genes produces a severe disease.

The haemoglobin molecule consists of haem groups and two different types of protein chains known as **globins**. In sickle cell disease there is a mutation of one DNA base in the gene on chromosome 11 which codes for one type of globin. Specifically, the DNA triplet code –CTC– changes to –CAC–.

This causes substitution of the wrong amino acid at a particular point in the globin chain, namely **valine** instead of **glutamic acid**. This small alteration changes the physical property of the haemoglobin molecule. In the presence of low oxygen concentrations sickle cell haemoglobin tends to polymerize into clumps which change the shape of the red blood cell, typically to a sickle shape. However, this only usually occurs when most of the haemoglobin is affected, as in those inheriting both abnormal genes. About half of the haemoglobin in the carriers is affected but the presence of normal haemoglobin inhibits polymer formation.

The abnormal red cells in sickle cell anaemia tend to clog up small blood vessels and cause tissue infarctions, which may involve bones and internal organs. Such attacks (**crises**) occur suddenly and are extremely painful. Patients also have **anaemia** (low level of haemoglobin in the blood) and are prone to bacterial infections. Events that often precipitate sickle cell crises are dehydration, infection, cold, exercise and pregnancy. Conditions of low oxygen pressure, as may occur at high altitude, or during some surgical procedures, are particularly dangerous for these patients. Carriers of the disease are not normally affected clinically, except in extreme circumstances of oxygen deprivation.

As yet, there is no cure for the disease but new types of treatment are under investigation. General supportive medical measures currently available in developed countries allow many patients to survive into middle age. In developing countries many patients with sickle cell anaemia die in early childhood.

Cystic fibrosis

Cystic fibrosis is an autosomal recessive disease that affects the lungs and the digestive system, especially the pancreas. It is one of the commonest single gene disorders of Caucasians, affecting one in every two thousand live births. Carriers of one cystic fibrosis gene are completely symptomless. There is no known advantage to the carrier state.

The defective gene, which is on chromosome 7, codes for a protein in the membrane of epithelial cells. Several mutations have been identified. The protein is normally a transporter of ions across membranes, probably chloride ions, and its activity affects water movement in various ducts. In cystic fibrosis there is abnormal salt and water transport which leads to an increased concentration of sodium chloride in the sweat, a diagnostic test for the condition. The abnormality also causes the mucus in various ducts to become excessively viscid or sticky, and it is this that gives rise to the disastrous clinical effects. The sticky mucus obstructs small ducts and encourages infection, particularly in the lungs.

Typically, cystic fibrosis presents in early childhood with repeated chest infections, impaired food absorption and retarded growth. The sticky mucus blocks the ducts of the pancreas which becomes damaged and is unable to supply digestive enzymes to the intestinal lumen. Poor digestion leads to the production of offensive fatty stools. A few years ago many patients died in childhood from extensive lung damage and infection. Now, with intensive supportive therapy, most patients are living well into adulthood, although other problems may then arise. As yet, there is no cure. Recent discoveries of the nature of the basic defect may offer some hope of finding a more specific form of treatment.

The management of genetic disorders

Clinical genetics is another medical specialism. The relevant clinical and laboratory services are based in a few highly specialised units.

Genetic counselling can be given when there is a family history of a genetic disorder. In such cases prospective parents can be advised on the chances of a pregnancy producing an affected child and on the options available to them. Accurate counselling requires accurate diagnosis of the condition in an affected member of the family. This involves careful clinical and laboratory investigation. For some disorders there are specific methods available for the analysis of the protein abnormality (e.g. enzyme deficiency) or even the defective

DNA. Modern techniques sometimes allow diagnosis in the fetus at an early stage of pregnancy. Prenatal (antenatal) diagnosis provides an opportunity to make an informed choice about the future of the pregnancy.

For some genetic diseases it is possible to test people for carrier status. Population screening has so far tended to be selective, concentrating on at-risk groups.

Apart from symptomatic relief, there is no effective treatment available for most genetic diseases. In a few the progress of the disease can be slowed or its effects reduced or even largely abolished. For instance, adequate and early correction of abnormal plasma phenylalanine levels by appropriate dietary manipulations can prevent the development of mental retardation in phenylketonuria. Haemophilia can be controlled by regular intravenous infusions of factor VIII. General modern medical measures can prolong and improve the lives of people with cystic fibrosis and sickle-cell anaemia. Attempts to replace missing enzymes by various manoeuvres in a number of diseases have had only limited success. In a few patients transplantation of compatible bone marrow from an unaffected sibling has cured thalassaemia.

Recent scientific advances have opened up new possibilities for the treatment of some genetic diseases, but it may be some time before research procedures can be reliably and safely transformed into routine clinical practices.

5
MIND AND DISEASE

Introduction

Cognition, mind and brain

Cognition is the mental process by which information or knowledge is acquired, stored and manipulated. The seat of human cognitive processes, such as learning, thinking, reasoning and memory, and of emotion and mood, is the brain. The 'mind' is an imprecise concept which refers in an abstract way to that part of us responsible for thought, feelings and the like. For our purposes it is more helpful to consider the individual mental processes and how they interact.

The analogy between computer information processing and human cognition has proved fruitful not only as a model for illustrating the interaction between subjectively abstract cognitive processes and the biological structures within the brain but also as a useful tool for advancing understanding of how human cognition may actually work. Obviously, computers and brains are made of different materials, are of different construction and use different types of signals to convey messages. The brain is much more complicated, but both are information processing systems that receive, interpret, store, retrieve and compare data, make decisions and initiate and control actions in peripheral devices. The material and structure of the brain, the hardware in computer terms, provides the machinery for the handling, storage and processing of information. Some new computer systems process sets of data in parallel and use so-called **neural networks** (not real nerves). Unlike the more traditional computer processors, in which single elements of data are examined rapidly one at a time, the newer innovations can process many items simultaneously. These advances have facilitated the development of systems that seek a degree or probability of likeness between large sets of data (e.g. comparing visual impressions of faces), rather than the more absolute pre-programmed match typically sought by the highly logical traditional computer. Such devices are capable of learning from experience. The process appears to be closely analogous to that used by the brain. The merging of knowledge and research in the fields of experimental psychology, neurobiology and computer science is helping to advance rapidly our understanding of how the brain works. This may be the next dramatic explosion in our knowledge of ourselves.

Damage to the hardware structure of the brain can produce gross effects such as the neurological deficits seen in stroke. The effects on communication and motor activity are fairly obvious because they are the interfaces with the outside world. But physical damage can also affect cognitive processes, behaviour and mood. At the other extreme, information from the outside world can sometimes have a profound effect on our mood and behaviour. Although this may sometimes cause a physical reaction in the body (e.g. autonomic responses), it does not cause gross physical change in the brain. Information might affect our cognitive or emotional state but it does not cause detectable neurological damage.

There is, however, an intermediary zone, a point at which the finer molecular aspects of brain structure interface with information, where the details of molecular activity determine information and vice versa. There are also biochemical systems that fine tune the levels of special chemicals (**neurotransmitters**) which transmit signals across the junctions between nerves; there are several such systems in the brain. Some mental illnesses, such as schizophrenia and major depression, may have both a **molecular** (**organic**) and **mental** (**functional** or

non-organic) basis, with many factors interacting to produce the final clinical effect.

Behaviour

Behaviour is the way we respond to things. Responses may be largely automatic, including acquired skills, such as many of the reactions involved in driving, or they may involve considerable deliberation. The stimuli prompting the response can originate from the outside world or from inside our brains. Human behaviour is largely learnt; it adapts so that the consequences of previous actions modify future responses, normally to advantage. Learning involves the storage of information in the memory. The newborn baby has an almost blank memory. In the first year or two the child explores objects and learns about their physical properties through the senses. Then it learns to put names to the objects. By five years the child has a vocabulary of some 2,000 words and is forming sentences. Motor skills must be learnt too. The brain develops a compendium of instructions for complex movements such as those required for walking, talking and manipulating objects. Specialised parts of the brain, such as the cerebellum, co-ordinate and fine tune the responses of the muscle groups, producing smoother and better controlled movements.

The childhood experience of interactions with other human beings has a considerable influence on personality in later life. Personality is the overall regular mode of behaviour that distinguishes and characterises individual people. Its final form generally emerges by the end of childhood and remains relatively stable in adult life. There may be a genetic component too. Some types of personality stand out more readily from the average, but they are not necessarily abnormal, it is very much a question of degree and what is acceptable to the peer group. Most of us would recognise the following types: a bit touchy, suspicious and doesn't like criticism; optimistic, sociable and takes risks; pessimistic, unsociable and moody. Extreme deviations of personality (**personality disorders**) may cause serious problems for the affected individual and for the people in contact with them.

Cognitive processes

Let us examine what happens when something in the environment stimulates our senses, for instance the sight of a particular object. The eye transmits a representation of the object to the brain. The brain's awareness of this sensory stimulus is **sensation**. The information may be incomplete, perhaps only part of the object was visible. The sensation is held briefly in the brain to allow comparisons with any similar but not necessarily identical images held in the memory stores. The object may or may not be recognised. **Perception** is the interpretation of the sensation, what we think we see. Expectations, fears, desires and previous experience can influence perception.

Illusions and **hallucinations** are abnormalities of perception. Illusion is a misinterpretation of a sensation arising from something in the outside world; the thing exists but the brain produces an impression of something different. An hallucination is a perception in the absence of an external stimulus; in other words the person sees or hears something that is not actually there in reality, although they may believe it to be real. Sensory images pass inappropriately from the memory stores to the processing areas responsible for perception, where they are perceived as being real. Hallucinations of sight and sound are the commonest. They are important in the diagnosis of mental illness but can occur in other conditions and occasionally even in healthy people.

There are several types of memory. We shall consider just a few aspects of sensory memory which is the record of our perceptions and the basis of our knowledge and experience. There is a short working memory which is not permanent but allows data of immediate interest to be processed. The processing unit transfers some information to a long-term memory system which provides a more robust molecular representation of the data, a more permanent record. The long-term memory can be divided into **recent memory** (e.g. remembering what you had for breakfast) and **remote memory** (e.g. important events in previous years). The placing of the record in the memory store is known as **registration** or **storage**. Copying the memory from the store to the processing unit is **retrieval**; the memory is not removed, just read, like a read only memory

(ROM) in a computer. **Re-call** is the conscious awareness of the retrieved memory. Fortunately we are not aware of most of the retrieval activities; only selected material filters into consciousness. An early and important abnormality in **dementia**, a progressive degeneration of mental function caused by brain disease, is an inability to remember new material. This causes impairment of recent memory but not remote memory.

Specific memories involving one sense, such as the visual representation of an object, are held in particular regions of the cerebral cortex. However, we often remember events which require the recall of complex visual and auditory (sound) perceptions, conversations, orientation in time and space and our emotional reaction at the time. The components of such memories are spread widely throughout the cortex.

Let us continue with our hypothetical scenario. Recognition of an object stimulates a search of the memory banks for previous experience of that object. The retrieved memories may come from different periods in a person's life, and they may bring with them additional, but associated, memory baggage. Perhaps on a recent occasion perception of the object was associated with some advantage. The reasoning processes might take all this into account and come to the conclusion that the present opportunity might also provide some advantage. But perhaps a shadowy memory from childhood is also lurking in the background, it might be retrieved but not necessarily recalled to consciousness in any detail. What was perceived as a similar object in childhood might at that time have been associated with some hurtful (or pleasant) experience. The association could even have been coincidental; the immature mind of the young child may have been unable to distinguish accurately between the events. Whatever the truth, the memory baggage might still cause unpleasant (or pleasurable) feelings without any apparent explanation. Some potentially hurtful or fearsome memories may be **repressed**, not normally allowed to come into consciousness at all. Their presence in the background may explain some anxiety states.

Personal beliefs and values, and perceptions of other people's attitudes, are also taken into account before we finally respond to a situation. We are often forced to strike attitudes without adequate knowledge, attitudes that may or may not be to our advantage, and may even be illogical given the full facts. These conflicts influence our behaviour throughout life.

Neurology, psychiatry and psychology

Neurologists are medically-qualified doctors who specialise in diseases of the nervous system that have a structural or biochemical (*organic*) basis. The patients may have physical and/or mental problems. Psychiatrists are medically-qualified doctors who specialise in the diagnosis and treatment of mental illness. Sometimes they see patients whose psychiatric symptoms are due to organic disease, but not usually the type of patient commonly seen by the neurologist. Crudely put, in computer jargon, we could call the neurologist the 'hardware' doctor and the psychiatrist the 'software' doctor. Each must know something of the other's subject, but they are very different disciplines requiring different knowledge, skills and approach.

Other hospital doctors and general practitioners see a wide range of conditions with physical and mental components. The compartmentalised training of doctors and the divisions in the practice of medicine sometimes allow patients to fall between the cracks. For instance, psychological problems in patients with physical brain disorders (e.g. stroke) may not always get adequate attention.

Psychologists study cognition and behaviour. Some use psychological methods to assist in the treatment of some psychiatric and psychological problems, for instance phobias and behavioural and learning difficulties. Psychotherapy encompasses a rather disparate group of specialised psychological techniques practised by different schools of therapists. Psychologists and psychotherapists are not usually medically qualified and do not prescribe drugs. The place of psychological therapies in the treatment of psychiatric disorders is discussed briefly on page 134.

Brain-body connections

Dozens of nerves arise from the brain and spinal cord (CNS) to form the peripheral nervous system. They contain large numbers of individual nerve fibres which distribute to all parts of the body. Motor nerves supply action signals to the muscles of the face, neck, trunk and limbs. There are different types of sensory receptors that relay information about the outside world to the brain. The obvious ones are those of the special senses responsible for vision, hearing, smell and taste. Specialised nerve endings in the skin respond to physical stimuli. Their signals are relayed to the brain to provide the sensations of touch, warmth, cold or pain. Sensory receptors in muscles and joints provide information about position and movement and are part of a feedback loop that ensures smooth, co-ordinated muscle action.

The cerebral cortex provides conscious awareness of our physical body: knowing one part from another, its orientation and position, distinguishing left from right, recognising our personal space and that beyond. Damage to particular areas, after stroke for example, can disrupt these faculties. Abnormal perceptions of body image occur in some forms of mental disorder. Patients with anorexia nervosa often believe they are fatter than they really are. People suffering from schizophrenia may have a distorted view of the boundary of self and non-self in terms of mental territory.

Another part of the peripheral nervous system is responsible for the automatic control of internal house-keeping operations, the regulation of major organs and systems. This is the **autonomic nervous system**. We are usually unaware of its activities and it is not normally amenable to voluntary control. Its functions include the control of blood pressure, blood flow to the tissues and organs, gastro-intestinal tract activities, sweating, salivary gland secretion and the size of the pupils (of the eye). It pervades almost every part of the body. Occasionally we are aware of its actions, for instance when nervousness causes a rapid heart beat, 'butterflies' in the stomach, a dry mouth, sweating and a frequent urge to pass urine. In fact, emotions such as joy, misery, anger and fear consist of two components, a mental response to the situation and an autonomic nervous system response which enhances the character and intensity of feeling.

Deep in the cranium, at the underside or base of the brain, towards the centre of the head, is a small but intricate area of brain known as the **hypothalamus**. It contains collections of neurons and tracts of nerve fibres which connect to many other specialised areas of the central nervous system, including the cerebral cortices. It plays a major role in the regulation and coordination of essential bodily functions and in **homeostasis**, the maintenance of the internal status quo in the face of a changing external environment. The hypothalamus integrates the activities of the autonomic nervous system. It is also involved in body temperature control, basic animal drives such as eating, drinking and sexual behaviour, and in emotional response. Furthermore, the hypothalamus also controls the **endocrine system**, a collection of glands that secrete hormones directly into the blood stream. These hormones control specific aspects of metabolism in the target tissues and organs.

The **pituitary gland** is a pea-sized structure lying immediately beneath the hypothalamus, to which it is connected by a short stalk. The hypothalamus controls the pituitary gland which in turn controls other endocrine glands such as the thyroid and adrenal cortex. Some hormones from the pituitary act directly on tissue metabolism; for instance, the antidiuretic hormone (ADH, vasopressin) acts on the kidney as described earlier (see page 42), growth hormone is necessary for normal body growth in childhood. The hypothalamus is itself influenced by levels of circulating hormones such as thyroid hormone from the thyroid gland and **cortisol** from the adrenal cortex. This provides an effective feedback control mechanism.

There are two **adrenal glands**. They are small structures which lie on top of the kidneys and have an excellent blood supply. The small core of the gland (the **medulla**) contains special cells producing the substance **adrenaline** which helps us cope with 'fight and flight' situations. The medulla is under the control of the autonomic nervous system. The **adrenal cortex**, the outer region of the gland, secretes steroid hormones into the blood stream. One of these is cortisol, also known as **hydrocortisone**. A specific pituitary hormone, namely **adrenocorticotrophic hormone** (**ACTH**), stimulates cortisol production in the adrenal cortex. The hypothalamus controls ACTH production in the pituitary. In normal circumstances plasma cortisol levels are highest in the morning. Some mental stress situations result in higher plasma cortisol levels, but the response is variable. Cortisol probably provides vital protection during episodes of severe physical stress, such as trauma, burns etc. However, although much is known about some of its effects on metabolism, its role and precise mode of action in stress situations is less well understood. One effect of high cortisol levels is to depress the immune response. There are suggestions that the brain may influence the general level of the immune response through this or some other mechanism.

In summary, a number of physical systems connect and integrate the activities of brain and body. The hypothalamus links and co-ordinates mental activities with the body's automatic control systems and is important for the maintenance of a stable internal environment.

Psychiatric disorders

Introduction

Disease can be difficult to define, and this is especially true in psychiatry. Spectacular and extreme abnormalities of behaviour may of course quite readily attract the label of mental illness, or even insanity. However, some of the symptoms of mental illness merge almost imperceptibly with normal responses to life. This is particularly true of the less severe forms of anxiety and depression. The diagnosis is easier when the symptoms are severe, incapacitating and seem to be out of proportion to, or bear little obvious relationship to, any external events which may have triggered the condition.

Even so, at any particular time about one-seventh of the populations of the UK and US are thought to be affected by some sort of mental disorder. The majority are cases of mild to moderate depression or anxiety. Up to a third of all patients attending general practice surgeries and general hospitals may have a mental disorder. At some time during their lives one per cent of the population will suffer from schizophrenia and probably more than five per cent will suffer from severe depressive illness. Mental illness is a major health problem throughout the world. And its management is costly.

The accurate diagnosis of mental illness requires skill and experience. Several interviews and the lapse of some time may be required before the true nature of the disease emerges. The psychiatrist will rigorously examine many facets of mental function such as mood, the nature of the patient's thoughts and thought processes, perception, ability to store, retrieve and associate data, and the patient's own insight into their condition. The patient's personality and background, including family and social history, are also taken into account. The initial diagnosis is made in terms of syndromes consisting of particular internationally-recognised combinations of clinical symptoms and signs (often called **phenomena** in psychiatry). The psychiatric assessment also attempts to identify any problems accentuating or arising from the condition that may require attention.

Causes

The causes of most forms of mental illness are not precisely known. Different schools of thought variously favour **organic factors** (structural, cellular or molecular brain abnormalities) and non-organic or **psychogenic factors** (those affecting the *mind*) as the most important underlying causes, depending on the type of disorder. The general consensus is that psychiatric disease is often caused by the interaction of multiple factors. Thus, there may be underlying causes, perhaps genetic influences and early childhood experiences, which make an individual particularly prone. Stressful circumstances in later life (e.g. bereavement, family crisis) may trigger the onset of the disease. Personality and sex may affect its presentation. Family and social tensions may help to perpetuate the condition in some cases.

Damage to brain structure can cause mental illness, with or without the assistance of psychogenic factors. It may be due to a specific genetic defect or one of a number of other processes affecting the brain (e.g. trauma, tumour, stroke, infection, degeneration). General chemical disturbances (e.g. hypoxia, hypoglycaemia, uraemia, alcoholism) may also affect brain function and cause acute impairment of the cognitive processes. Blatant organic brain disorders such as these can produce a variety of mental disturbances, including symptoms seen in psychiatric syndromes such as major depression and schizophrenia. The stress caused by the disease also contributes to the overall mental condition. Anxiety and depression commonly occur in dementias such as Alzheimer's disease. Indeed anxiety and depression are common accompaniments of many illnesses, physical as well as mental.

Genetic factors operate in schizophrenia and severe depressive illness but they are not straightforward and may involve the interaction of multiple genes. This, together with the discovery of subtle abnormalities of brain biochemistry, and the corresponding specific chemical actions of certain drugs that provide relief, suggest an organic basis, particularly in schizophrenia.

Psychogenic (i.e. psychological) factors are thought to be important in the development of depression, but less so in schizophrenia. Psychogenic factors are also particularly important in anxiety disorders. Reiteration of abnormal thoughts and perceptions may further reinforce false ideas. A severely depressed person may become increasingly preoccupied with ideas of worthlessness and hopelessness. Schizophrenics may develop strange behaviours in response to their perception of events in an apparently bizarre world.

Classification of mental illness by cause or disease process is not yet possible. Only rarely in an individual case can the major causative factor be identified with some certainty. Exceptions are some of the clear cut organic disorders but these comprise a minute fraction of the psychiatric workload. Also, diseases with different causes may present with similar phenomena (symptoms and signs).

Diagnostic labels

An accurate diagnosis is just as important in psychiatry as it is in other branches of medicine. It allows the possibility of providing the most effective treatment and giving the best advice. To some extent this is hampered by the lack of knowledge of the causes of mental illness and the nature of the disease processes involved. Even the division into organic and non-organic diseases is blurred. The use of descriptive labels that are meaningful and of practical value is of prime importance.

The term **psychosis** is frequently applied to severe psychiatric disorders in which the patient has a distorted contact with reality and poor insight into their condition. These phenomena can occur, although not invariably, in schizophrenia, severe depressive illness and some forms of organic brain disease. **Neurosis** is a label often applied to non-psychotic mental disorders such as anxiety states and less severe forms of depression in which insight is generally preserved. Many psychiatrists now frown upon the classification of mental illnesses into simple categories such as organic, psychotic and neurotic disorders.

Modern psychiatric diagnosis follows guidelines developed by the World Health Organisation and the American Psychiatric Association. The following account is necessarily sketchy and belies the comprehensive nature of these initiatives. Typical disease categories are **organic disorders** (which includes **dementia**), **schizophrenia**, **mood disorders** (which includes **depression** and **mania**) and **anxiety disorders**. There are several others. The disease categories are clinical syndromes consisting of particular collections of phenomena. Diagnosis is based on probability rather than certainty, with some phenomena having more significance than others. The following notes illustrate some of the typical features of selected syndromes.

Dementia

Dementia is a collective term for a chronic degenerative brain syndrome in which there is progressive loss of mental functions. Senile dementia is relatively common in old age and is usually due to Alzheimer's disease or vascular disease, or both. Dementia in middle age is uncommon but may be caused by the above conditions and many others (including Huntington's chorea, alcoholism and AIDS). The cause of Alzheimer's disease is not known; there are characteristic degenerative changes in the brain. Prominent early features of dementia are loss of recent memory and mood changes. Later there may be marked deterioration of intellectual ability, anti-social behaviour and a coarsening of the personality.

Schizophrenia

Schizophrenia is one of the most serious forms of mental illness, its effects can be devastating. Literally, schizophrenia means 'split mind', but it is not the dual personality of popular fiction. It is a disruption of the thought processes which leads to ideas and behaviours that seem strange and inexplicable to other people. The condition usually first appears in early adult life. It may take several forms and the severity and course of the disease varies. Some patients have an acute attack and then recover completely, others have recurrent attacks, and some suffer a relentless downhill course.

The syndrome typically involves abnormalities of thought, perception and mood. Patients may believe that their thoughts are coming from some external agent, or are being transmitted to others. They may have beliefs that are clearly false and inappropriate when their background is taken into account (delusions). There may be abnormal connections between concepts, leading to illogical thought and incoherent statements. Auditory hallucinations may occur, typically in the form of voices commenting on the patient in the third person, or hearing thoughts spoken aloud. The patient's emotional responses may appear inappropriate to the circumstances. In the more chronic phases of the disease there may be social withdrawal, lack of motivation, apathy and a flattened emotional response to stimulating situations.

Mood disorders

Depression is common and occurs more frequently in women. It may be severe and associated with a lack of insight into the problems of the disease, or may be of a less severe nature. The typical features of severe depression are an abnormally depressed mood most of the day, general loss of interest, feelings of worthlessness, helplessness, hopelessness and guilt, and thoughts of death. Physical symptoms are often present in depression and these may be the main complaint when seeking medical advice. They include sleep disturbances, headaches, fatigue, constipation, anorexia, weight changes and reduced interest in sex.

Some patients prone to depressive illness also suffer from episodes of **mania** in which the mood is abnormally elevated, the opposite of depression. Symptoms then include elation, inflated self-esteem, streams of ideas with thoughts jumping about, fast speech, and a tendency towards behavioural excesses and indiscretions. Patients who suffer both extremes of mood, depression on one occasion and mania on another, are said to have a **bipolar affective disorder** (previously called manic-depressive psychosis).

The outlook for patients with depressive illness is generally good with the assistance of modern psychiatric treatment. The possibility of suicide in severe depression must always be borne in mind.

Anxiety disorders

Anxiety is a normal response to threat. It consists of psychological distress (e.g. worrying) and arousal, a stimulating effect of the autonomic nervous system. When the emotion of anxiety is excessive and inappropriate to the circumstances, or abnormally prolonged, it may be very distressing or even crippling. Abnormal anxiety reactions may be generalised, for instance, a **free-floating anxiety** unconnected with anything in particular, or specific, as in the case of the **phobias** in which there is irrational excessive fear of a particular type of thing such as spiders, mice, heights, flying, closed spaces, public places etc. As well as the psychological symptoms, such as apprehension and a fear of impending disaster, anxiety disorders are accompanied by bodily reactions such as muscular tensions, headaches, trembling hands, sweating, palpitations, dizziness, breathlessness, dry mouth and diarrhoea. Anxiety often accompanies other psychiatric disorders.

Learning disability

This is the term often used in the UK for the condition previously known as mental retardation. It generally refers to the situation in which a person's intellectual functioning is, and usually always has been, impaired to the extent that they need support to help them cope with everyday living. There are problems with names and definitions. Some authoritative bodies still use the label mental retardation. The Mental Health Act of 1983 (England) used the terms mental handicap and mental impairment, the latter being reserved for individuals who also have problematical behaviour and may require compulsory detention in a hospital. Some people feel that labels such as handicap and retardation stigmatise the affected individuals, tend to limit our expectations of them and influence policies aimed at them as a group. People with learning disability may have an impaired problem-solving ability but not necessarily an impaired memory. They may have other problems too, mental or physical, depending on the cause of their condition.

Traditionally, the degree of intellectual impairment has been measured using specially designed intelligence tests. A score (IQ, intelligence quotient) of 100 represents an average intelligence. A score of less than 70 is often taken as an indicator of mental handicap. Medical causes of learning disability, such as chromosome and genetic abnormalities, are often present in the more severely affected (e.g. IQ less than 50). Some individuals with lesser degrees of disability represent the lower end of the normal range of ability. The ability and behaviour of the individual are dependent on more than just IQ.

In terms of professional vocation and practice, learning disability has generally been a specialist subject separate from mainstream psychiatry.

Alcohol misuse

Substance misuse may be regarded as substance taking that could have adverse medical or social effects. It applies to alcohol, tobacco, drugs and other substances. Misuse may be sporadic, as in the occasional alcoholic binge, or regular. Chronic misuse can lead to **dependence**, a state in which a person has a compulsion to continue taking the substance because of the need to experience its effects and/or to avoid unpleasant withdrawal symptoms. Dependence can be physical and/or mental, the pattern and extent depending on the substance. We shall consider only alcohol, but the principles apply to several substances.

Alcohol availability, cultural factors and psychosocial pressures influence drinking patterns and contribute to dependence in susceptible people. A genetic tendency and psychiatric disorders may be predisposing factors in a few, but there is little evidence that these factors are important in the majority of people who develop alcohol dependence. Chronic alcohol consumption leads to **tolerance**, a state in which increasingly large amounts are required to satisfy the need. This results from homeostatic biochemical adjustments in response to the repeated drug challenge. Some of the typical features of alcohol dependence are: increased tolerance to the intoxicating effects of alcohol; drinking becomes the priority activity, to the detriment of the drinker and their family; the repertoire of drinking becomes narrower; regular withdrawal symptoms, which are relieved by further drinking.

Apart from the obvious disastrous social consequences, chronic excessive alcohol consumption can cause psychological reactions (e.g. depression, jealousy, violence), withdrawal symptoms and a vast number of serious medical and psychiatric disorders. At first the withdrawal symptoms typically consist of a feeling of agitation and a generalised rapid tremor in the morning, a few hours after the last drink. Later they may involve severe and sometimes dangerous neurological and psychiatric reactions. Other clinical aspects of excessive alcohol consumption are considered in chapter eight, page 180.

———— **Psychiatric treatment** ————

Psychiatric treatment includes psychological techniques, drugs and occasionally electroconvulsive therapy (ECT).

Psychological treatments

Typical psychological treatments are supportive therapy, interpretive psychotherapy, behaviour therapy and cognitive therapy. Therapy sessions may be one-to-one or involve groups of people and they are usually led by professionals with specialised training, not necessarily doctors. Supportive therapy essentially consists of the kind of counselling that should occur to some extent during any consultation. It involves empathy, getting the patient to air their problems and worries, listening and giving credible explanations, advice and reassurance. It increases the patient's trust, confidence and co-operation, and it can have a positive therapeutic effect, often enhancing the benefits of other forms of treatment.

Interpretive psychotherapy (psychoanalysis) is a lengthy, and therefore often expensive, form of treatment which attempts to identify repressed fears and memories and to modify the psychological conflicts arising from them. The methods are very specialised and most therapists undergo extensive training. There are different schools of psychotherapy with different approaches. Psychoanalysis can only be used for certain types of disorder, such as anxiety states and mild depression; it is contraindicated in psychosis. The **behaviour therapies** aim to modify abnormal behaviour by altering the individual's response to relevant stimuli or situations (e.g. phobias). **Cognitive therapy** attempts to identify negative patterns of thinking (e.g. hopelessness, worthlessness), to help the patient understand how such thought patterns affect behaviour and to substitute more positive thinking patterns.

Drug therapy

Modern drug therapy can be highly effective in relieving the distressing symptoms of serious mental illness. Sometimes high doses are required to control the conditions. Side effects can be a problem. Three important groups of drugs used in psychiatry are neuroleptics, antidepressants and anxiolytics. **Neuroleptics** are antipsychotic drugs used in the treatment of schizophrenia. They can relieve symptoms such as hallucinations, delusions and thought disorder and convert many acutely ill patients to normal activity. **Antidepressants** produce satisfactory responses in the majority of patients with depression but benefit is not apparent until after at least two to three weeks on the treatment. The length of treatment required varies considerably. **Anxiolytics** are commonly known as tranquillisers. They can be effective for the short-term treatment of severe or crippling anxiety (e.g. two to four week course). Unfortunately, longer treatments with these drugs can lead to a state of psychological and physical dependency. Great care must be taken when withdrawing patients from psychiatric drug therapy because of the possibility of severe withdrawal reactions. This should be done under medical supervision.

Electroconvulsive therapy (ECT)

Electroconvulsive therapy appears drastic and crude, but it can be the most effective treatment in some patients with severe psychotic depression, especially when there is a high risk of suicide. The patient is anaesthetised and a brief electric current is applied across the head. A drug is given to relax the muscles and prevent damage due to convulsion. Conducted properly it is generally a safe procedure.

– Physical disease and mental state –

There is no doubt that the mental state can influence health and the response to disease and treatment. But claims that psychological factors are major underlying causes of many serious physical diseases such as hypertension, peptic ulcer, asthma and cancer have not generally found favour: there is, so far, little convincing scientific evidence. Stress and anxiety certainly contribute to some major illnesses and may be responsible for some less serious but nevertheless troublesome conditions. Stress appears to be one of the factors associated with coronary thrombosis in the type of personality that strives aggressively to compete and overachieve in a challenging work environment. Stress may sometimes precipitate angina or fatal arrhythmias (abnormal heart rhythms) in patients with pre-existing heart disease. Anxiety is high during severe asthma attacks and its persistence may contribute to exhaustion and deterioration.

Anxiety and depression can affect internal bodily functions and cause a variety of physical disturbances and symptoms which may lead patients to believe that they have serious physical illness. Chronic mental stress may be accompanied by undesirable patterns of muscular tension and posture which may in turn produce troublesome physical symptoms.

Some people complain vehemently about a variety of symptoms, or are convinced about the presence of a particular disease, and yet the doctor can find no evidence of a physical abnormality. Very occasionally a striking dysfunction of a part of the body may occur, such as blindness, paralysis or memory loss, for which there is no obvious physical explanation. Many of these people have a history of emotional problems and disturbed relationships, and some suffer from depression. These phenomena may represent an expression of psychological stress. The close attention given by the carers often reinforces the behaviour pattern. These conditions can be difficult to treat. Obviously, great care must be taken to exclude the possibility of physical disease as the cause.

Physical disease in general is often accompanied by a noticeable psychological reaction, usually anxiety followed by depression. The latter normally resolves when the patient recovers. Additional psychogenic factors that can intensify or prolong depression are the unwelcome lifestyle and social changes that sometimes accompany or follow serious illness. The viral infections influenza, glandular fever and hepatitis are often followed by a prolonged period of depression, which may have an *organic* element.

Pain

Pain is one of the most important subjects in medicine. It is a key feature of diagnosis and arguably the major cause of fear and suffering in patients. And yet it is poorly understood and sometimes badly managed. Pain has a mental and physical basis. We recognise it easily enough, and much is known about its biology and psychology, but scientifically and philosophically it is difficult to define. Pain is an unpleasant sensation with an emotional component. It generally arises from stimuli capable of producing tissue damage and has an obvious protective function in normal circumstances. We very quickly learn to avoid potentially painful situations. Here we shall review briefly the physical and mental factors that influence the phenomenon of pain. Particular medical aspects are discussed in other chapters, pages 142, 202 and 216.

Tissue injury stimulates the generation of signals in local nerve endings. The signals pass along the peripheral sensory nerve fibres and enter the central nervous system (CNS) at the corresponding anatomical level. For instance, those from the leg go to the lower part of the spinal cord. Signals from peripheral fibres subserving the sensation of pain stimulate cells in the spinal cord that regulate and generate the next set of signals in the pain pathway. The latter signals are relayed to the brain for further processing.

Although the brain is necessary to experience pain, there is no single specific pain centre. The intensity of pain depends on how many signals reach the relevant brain areas. This in turn depends on the rate at which signals pass from the peripheral nerve fibres into the CNS and on the extent to which those signals are then relayed in subsequent pain pathways to higher levels. There are neurological 'gates' in the CNS which control the flow of signals at different levels and therefore ultimately the number entering the higher brain centres responsible for conscious appreciation of pain. Stimulation of certain peripheral nerve fibres can close down particular CNS gates, which reduces the flow of signals and therefore the amount of pain experienced. Gates may close at higher levels in response to stress, suggestion and the **placebo effect** (a beneficial effect arising from the belief that an agent will be effective even though there is no specific biological reason why it should be). Anxiety can actually increase the experience of pain. A number of psychological measures can help patients to cope with pain. Optimum control of chronic pain sometimes requires **multiple convergent therapy**, in which drug treatment, nerve stimulation methods and psychological techniques are combined.

6

DIAGNOSIS

The diagnostic process

Diagnosis is the identification of the patient's disease. The diagnostic process has two stages, data gathering and data interpretation. The accuracy of the diagnosis depends on the sufficiency and quality of the information obtained during the clinical interview and subsequent investigations. The doctor must judge how far to go to obtain the relevant information. Diagnosis sometimes requires an extensive clinical examination and many special tests. Often it requires just a short interview with the patient, and no high-tech investigations.

The data needed to make a diagnosis come from the history, the physical examination and the investigations (tests). The **history** is the story of the complaint as told by the patient, or sometimes by other people such as the relatives. Key items that emerge from the history are the **symptoms**, the sensations or bodily changes experienced by the patient that provide evidence for the existence of a disease. Common symptoms are pain, nausea, vomiting, diarrhoea, constipation, cough, abnormal bleeding, breathlessness, weakness, tiredness and changes in appetite, weight, mood and bodily functions. The **physical examination** is a systematic examination of the body in which the doctor uses his or her eyes, ears and hands (and occasionally sense of smell) to actively seek physical evidence of disease. A piece of evidence from the physical examination that supports the existence of a disease is called a **sign**.

After an initial assessment of the symptoms and signs the doctor may make a provisional diagnosis and then organise some special investigations, such as blood tests and X-rays. At this stage special tests may help to confirm or exclude the presence of particular conditions. Hospital doctors tend to take detailed histories, perform very thorough physical examinations and, often, organise several special investigations. For the majority of patients attending a general practice clinic such a comprehensive approach is generally not required, and may be quite inappropriate. A busy NHS general practitioner has only a few minutes available for each patient and must therefore adopt an efficient and focused approach to diagnosis.

The doctor interprets and evaluates the gathered evidence and produces a **differential diagnosis**. This is a list of the diseases which possibly could be responsible for the findings, starting with the most likely. Sometimes a less likely diagnosis in the list may be a medically more serious condition and may require specific investigation, if only to prove its absence. The process by which the average doctor arrives at his or her final diagnosis often seems arbitrary. The mental processes are complicated. In fact, the most probable diagnoses often come to mind during the first couple of minutes of the interview. The skilled clinician will modify the procedure economically in order to focus on and further verify the main diagnosis, and yet not neglect the possibility of a less likely but perhaps more sinister condition.

Diagnosis ultimately requires an evaluation of probability, the likelihood that a symptom, sign or test result, or a combination, indicates a particular disease. This requires a knowledge of how often the symptom, sign or test result occurs in that disease and how often the disease and the abnormal finding occur in general. Not surprisingly, computers are occasionally used for diagnostic decision-making. Given *all* the data, they can make more accurate predictions of diagnosis than many clinicians. However, experienced senior clinicians generally compete reasonably well, even without all the statistical information, much of which is not readily available in practice. They draw on years of clinical experience and an extensive knowledge of disease patterns. Thus, at times diagnosis may seem almost intuitive, an art rather than a science. However, there are circumstances when a computerised approach to diagnosis is highly desirable, for instance when probabilities arising from certain combinations of features can sway important decisions on the future management of the patient.

Symptoms and signs often point to the anatomical location of the disease, perhaps in a particular organ or tissue. This can considerably narrow down the number of possible diagnoses. Special investigations may be required to locate the lesion more precisely, to determine the extent of spread of the disease and to reveal or confirm its nature or cause. A single disease may produce several symptoms and signs, and this greatly assists diagnosis. Occasionally multiple findings are due to the presence of more than one disorder, particularly in the elderly.

Accurate diagnosis requires good clinical data. Even a computer cannot help with clinical decision-making if it is fed with unreliable information. A large and important part of the training of medical students and doctors involves the development of the skills necessary to elicit symptoms and signs accurately.

The history

The importance of the medical history cannot be overemphasised. The diagnosis can often be made from this alone; the physical examination and investigations may provide additional confirmation. Patients can assist the process of diagnosis considerably by thinking carefully about their symptoms before they see the doctor:

- when did the symptom first occur?
- where does it appear, or which part of the body seems to be affected?
- what is its nature and severity?
- how long does it last?
- how frequently does it occur?
- when did it last occur?

- is it associated with any particular events, or other symptoms?
- is it made worse or better by particular activities?

A concise to-the-point summary of events is most helpful. A rambling and inaccurate account distracts the doctor and uses up valuable time. Not unreasonably, patients often form their own opinion about the diagnosis before they attend the clinic, and sometimes they are right, particularly when a well-known complication occurs in a chronic condition for which they are already under medical care. However, there are potential problems. The doctor must form his or her own opinion from the symptoms. Human nature tends to colour our perceptions. Having thought of a diagnosis the patient may unwittingly modify the emphasis or description of the symptoms accordingly, which may be misleading. Even doctors occasionally do this when they are convinced about a diagnosis. The important point is that the symptoms should be described as accurately and objectively as possible.

The doctor will structure the interview according to the situation. However, there is a conventional format for a complete medical history. Initially the patient will be invited to give details of the present complaint, its past history, and any past or present treatment taken for it. The doctor will usually document the relevant events in chronological order. He or she will intervene now and then to confirm or amplify certain points. This may be followed by a more direct form of questioning to ascertain details of past medical history (other illnesses, operations, hospitalisations, immunisations, medicines, allergies, etc.), family history (genetic disorders, longevity, major illnesses and causes of death in relatives, especially parents, grandparents and siblings), social history where relevant and details of smoking habits and alcohol consumption. There will also be a series of questions designed to detect problems in various organs and systems. Women may be asked about their menstrual, contraceptive and reproductive histories.

Pain

Symptoms provide important clues to diagnosis but a good deal of knowledge and experience is often required to solve the puzzle correctly. The analysis of pain provides a good example.

Figure 6.1 indicates some of the diseases of internal organs that can give rise to pain in the midline at the front of the chest and abdomen. The list is not complete and some minor conditions may also cause pain in these regions. The distribution of the pain gives a clue to the site of the disease, although there is some overlap. Thus, a myocardial infarction typically causes pain behind the breastbone (**retrosternal pain**) and a peptic ulcer typically causes pain in the upper part of the abdomen below the breastbone (**epigastric pain**). However, sometimes a peptic ulcer causes retrosternal pain and myocardial infarction an epigastric pain. Pain often extends beyond the main site (**radiation**); this is a valuable diagnostic clue, but not necessarily very specific. In angina and myocardial infarction the chest pain may extend into the arms and neck, especially down the inside of the left arm. There are many conditions (not shown) that cause pain on the left or right sides of the trunk, rather than in the midline. In some instances the pain extends to the midline. Inflammation of the gall bladder (**cholecystitis**) causes pain in the right upper quadrant of the abdomen and sometimes in the epigastric region. An acute kidney infection may produce a pain in the loin that radiates down to the lower front abdominal wall. In acute appendicitis the pain often starts vaguely in the centre of the abdomen before it localises characteristically in the right lower quadrant.

Pain is sometimes referred to a site quite remote from the lesion. The usual cause of shoulder pain is damage or inflammation affecting tissues in the region of the joint. However, very occasionally, pain in the shoulder may be due to other causes such as irritation of the diaphragm caused by disease in the adjacent lung and pleura above or by leakage from a perforated peptic ulcer below. This is because the nerve supply to the diaphragm originates at the same spinal level as that supplying the shoulder. This is just one example of the phenomenon of **referred pain**. It is, for the unwary, and the untrained, a potential cause of serious misdiagnosis.

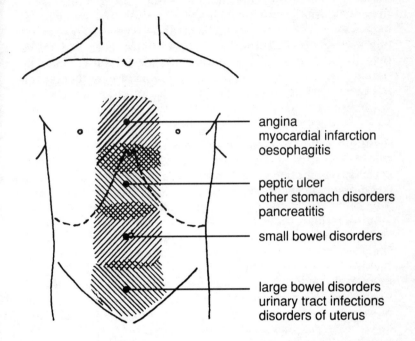

angina
myocardial infarction
oesophagitis

peptic ulcer
other stomach disorders
pancreatitis

small bowel disorders

large bowel disorders
urinary tract infections
disorders of uterus

Figure 6.1 Some causes of anterior midline trunk pain

Other characteristics of pain that assist in diagnosis are its quality, severity and duration (e.g. the persistent severe oppressive crushing ache of myocardial infarction), its timing (e.g. peptic ulcer pain often occurs around 2 a.m.) and whether or not anything relieves or aggravates it (e.g. food often relieves peptic ulcer pain; exertion or large meals may precipitate angina). The combination of pain with other symptoms further narrows down the possibilities.

The physical examination

Inexperienced medical students generally complete the history before proceeding with the physical examination. Experienced clinicians start to examine the patient as soon as they enter the surgery and continue to do so while they are taking the history. Initially this involves unobtrusive observations of demeanour, movement, speech, attitude, general appearance and any special features visible on the face, neck and hands (which sometimes provide valuable diagnostic clues). Once the patient has told his or her story the clinician may then examine them more actively, and continue the questioning. The rest of the examination is tailored to the situation and may concentrate mainly on one part or system.

A full physical examination includes a detailed assessment of the cardiovascular system, respiratory system, abdomen, breasts, lymphatic system and nervous system. If an abdominal problem is suspected, or is to be excluded, the doctor may also carry out a manual internal examination of the rectum (and sometimes the vagina). The order and style of the physical examination depend to some extent on the problem and on the preferences of the practitioner. It often tends to start from the head and work downwards. Consideration is usually given to patient comfort by limiting the number of changes of position. Thus, when examining the front of the chest the clinician may be gathering information on several systems simultaneously (e.g. cardiovascular and respiratory systems, and breasts). The procedures are not usually painful, although there may be some discomfort. It may be necessary to gently probe a painful area in order to determine more precisely the nature and site of a lesion, in the abdomen for example. The ambience and the bedside manner of the clinician are undoubtedly important in allaying anxiety and embarrassment. A patient should expect privacy and consideration. There is no excuse for leaving a person lying naked on the examination couch unnecessarily. However, clothes can considerably hamper a physical examination. Most clinicians manage to keep their patient's private areas discretely covered until they actually need to be examined. There is no reason why, if they so wish, a patient should not have a chaperon present during the examination. Indeed, some male doctors insist on this when examining women, and particularly when performing internal examinations. An interesting twist is that some patients insist on the right not to have a chaperon.

The traditional methods of the physical examination are inspection, palpation, percussion and auscultation. All four techniques may be used when examining the chest and abdomen. We shall briefly consider each method in turn. The number of possible signs that they may elicit is vast and this book cannot possibly do justice to this very technical subject. **Inspection** refers to careful observation with the eyes. This is partly accomplished while taking the history, as indicated previously, but there are particular items that must be checked during the systematic examination. This includes looking for abnormal or unusual colours, structures, contours or movements. The examiner may specifically inspect the eyes, ears, nose or throat using special devices, such as the **otoscope** which allows inspection of the external ear (that is from the outside to the ear drum) and the **ophthalmoscope** to visualise the retina at the back of the eye.

Palpation is the examination of a part of the body using the sense of touch. The fingers can be used to determine the size, shape, texture, attachments or movements of structures in or beneath the body surfaces (e.g. lumps, vessels, accessible organs) and to locate and characterise tenderness (e.g. due to an inflamed internal organ). Palpation can detect enlargement of the liver, spleen and kidneys.

Percussion is the delivery of a short sharp (but painless) tap to a surface or structure. The doctor may use his or her fingers in this way to detect abnormal density, for instance excess fluid surrounding the lung. It is rather like tapping barrels and tanks to determine where the liquid ends and the air begins. Solid tissues and collections of fluid produce a dull note whereas air produces a hollow resonance. A special hammer (with a rubber head) is sometimes used to percuss tendons in order to elicit certain types of nerve-muscle responses (tendon reflexes).

Auscultation is the technique of listening to sounds arising from inside the body, usually with an instrument called a **stethoscope**. Originally physicians placed their ear on the body surface. The stethoscope provides a more convenient method whereby the observer's ear is separated from the patient by a length of tubing. The various attachments at the patient end assist in listening to different types of noise. The sounds arise from mechanical vibrations inside the body, particularly those caused by the closure of the heart valves and the turbulent flow of liquids and gases.

Heart sounds are heard at the front of the chest. Normally two different sounds occur with each heart beat, one after the other. They are the **first heart sound**, which is due to closure of the mitral and tricuspid valves (the atrio-ventricular valves), and the **second heart sound**, which is due to closure of the aortic and pulmonary valves (the outlet valves). The reader may wish to refer to the section on the cardiac cycle in chapter two, see page 26. The first sound may be described as 'lub', and the second sound, which is shorter and of higher pitch, as 'dup'. Thus, the normal heart will produce the following sequence of noises:

.....lub...dup.....lub...dup.....lub...dup.....

The interval between 'lub' and 'dup' is **systole**, the period during which the heart expels blood into the main arteries. The interval between 'dup' and 'lub' is **diastole**, the period during which the ventricles relax and receive blood from the atria. Sometimes turbulent blood flow through the heart valves produces additional noises in the gaps between the heart sounds. These are **murmurs**, and they are either systolic murmurs or diastolic murmurs. There are other sounds too. Abnormal sounds and murmurs are important in the diagnosis of heart disease (e.g. valve disorders, congenital heart disease).

Auscultation is also used to detect abnormal air flow in different parts of the lung. The presence and nature of various crackles and wheezes and the character of sound conduction in the chest (after saying 'ninety-nine' for instance) provide important clues in the diagnosis of lung disorders. Stethoscopes can also be used to detect sounds of diagnostic interest in the abdomen, such as those arising from gas and fluid movement in the bowels (bowel sounds) and the heart beat of the fetus in the womb.

The examination of the nervous system involves a series of tests designed to elicit physical signs of neurological dysfunction. A particular combination of neurological signs, and a good knowledge of clinical neuroanatomy, often enables the doctor to pinpoint the position of the lesion, even to a specific part of the brain.

Internal digital (finger) examinations of the back passage (anus and rectum) and the vagina involve gentle palpation in order to detect abnormalities in or around these organs. The examiner's fingers are covered with a thin plastic glove to which a lubricant jelly is usually applied to ease access and reduce discomfort. One finger is used to examine the rectum; one or two fingers may be used to examine the vagina. These procedures may detect abnormal structures (e.g. enlarged prostate, carcinoma of the rectum) and tenderness (e.g. due to an abscess in the pelvis). Afterwards the doctor will inspect the glove for the presence of abnormal bleeding or discharge.

Vital signs

The medical examination generally includes an assessment of pulse, blood pressure and respiration. These so-called vital signs are often very helpful in diagnosis. They are also monitored regularly in many seriously ill patients and in these circumstances may provide valuable warnings of dangerous clinical situations.

Two important properties of the pulse are its rhythm and rate. One or both may be abnormal in heart disease – this will be considered in more detail in the next chapter (see page 155) when we consider electrocardiography. Conditions in which the pulse may be excessively rapid include exertion, anxiety, fever (raised temperature), heart disease, heavy loss of blood (e.g. from a bleeding peptic ulcer), thyrotoxicosis, anaemia and the administration of certain drugs (e.g. some of those used to treat asthma). The demonstration of a rapid pulse during sleep helps to exclude anxiety (and of course exertion) as a cause.

After severe blood loss the heart rate increases in an attempt to maintain the cardiac output and ensure an adequate perfusion of blood in vital tissues. The autonomic nervous system mediates the adjustments. If more than about 15 per cent of the blood volume is lost rapidly the cardiovascular system may then be unable to compensate adequately and the signs of shock may appear. Shock is due to inadequate perfusion of the tissues and organs. There are other causes apart from blood loss. It may occur after myocardial infarction if there is a fall in cardiac output due to a failing pump. Typical signs of shock are a rapid pulse and a low blood pressure. Severe or persistent shock is very dangerous and must be treated immediately.

—— Ancient and modern methods ——

Despite the great advances that have been made in many areas of medicine, a detached observer might be forgiven for thinking that some of the diagnostic procedures still used by doctors are a little anachronistic. Palpation and percussion are relatively crude methods, generally only allowing the detection of fairly gross changes. The oft-displayed stethoscope is hardly the flagship of modern medical science and technology. Considerable training is required to develop acceptable levels of skill and competence in physical examination. Some doctors become exquisitely expert in particular aspects, such as auscultation of the heart. In practice these traditional methods often provide a rapid and effective initial diagnostic screen, and sometimes nothing more is required. The medical profession tends to be conservative and is generally reluctant to abandon well tried and tested methods. Experience has often reinforced the wisdom of this approach. Nevertheless, new techniques and processes are always under investigation and those offering distinct advantages will, once proven, find their way into routine medical practice.

7

INVESTIGATIONS

Introduction

Special procedures that assist diagnosis but do not form part of the regular history and physical examination are known as investigations, or commonly as 'tests'. They are also used to assess general health status, organ function and response to treatment. Investigations include such things as X-rays, electrocardiography and tests on body tissues and fluids. They all require equipment. General practitioners commonly perform electrocardiography and simple tests on urine (e.g. for the presence of glucose, protein or blood). Other investigations may require the expertise and facilities of specialised hospital departments, some of which provide services for patients referred by their general practitioners as well as for hospital in-patients and out-patients.

Sometimes a few days pass by before the result of a test becomes available. There are a number of justifiable reasons for this. Some tests actually take time to perform properly. Investigations requiring very specialised laboratory procedures and those that are not in great demand may only be performed at intervals, perhaps once a week; to do them more frequently might overstrain limited resources and not be cost-effective. For certain types of test an expert opinion may be required to interpret the results accurately. The relevant hospital specialist may only be available to review such results at certain times. In general, procedures are tailored as far as possible to match the urgency of particular clinical situations.

Over the last few years there has been an explosion in the number of special tests available and in their technological sophistication. Used judiciously they can be a tremendous asset. The experienced clinician is usually very selective in his or her choice of investigations. At times there has been a vogue for using a large battery of tests to screen patients, partly because it happened to be technologically easy to do so. Occasionally this approach will detect an unsuspected and clinically important abnormality. However, it also gives rise to a number of apparently abnormal test results which may have little clinical relevance and can lead to further unnecessary investigation, anxiety and even longer stays in hospital. For a number of reasons, tests are sometimes fallible.

—— The Pathology Department ——

Pathology encompasses a number of specialist disciplines which in the larger hospitals, especially teaching hospitals, have their own separate departments, consultants and staff. The four main branches are **histopathology** (also known as morbid anatomy), **haematology**, **clinical chemistry** (also known as chemical pathology) and **microbiology**.

Histopathologists are the doctors who conduct post-mortems. But there is much more to this discipline. Tissues sometimes need to be examined by special microscopic techniques, a subject known as histology. This may be part of the post-mortem investigation, perhaps to determine the cause of death, or it may be part of the diagnostic process. For instance, histological examination of a breast lump and the corresponding local lymph nodes removed at operation can determine the nature of the tumour (benign, malignant, type of carcinoma etc.) and the extent of spread. It is a vital part of the grading and staging of malignant tumours (see chapter three, page 68). Precise diagnosis of liver and kidney disease sometimes necessitates removal of a tiny piece of the organ (**biopsy**) for histological examination. A related field is **cytology**, in which cells are examined for abnormalities (e.g. cells in cervical smear specimens).

The haematology laboratory provides tests for the investigation of blood cell disorders and clotting and bleeding abnormalities. The clinical chemistry laboratory analyses specific chemical components in human specimens, mainly plasma and urine. The microbiology department grows and/or identifies micro-organisms from patients' specimens (e.g. blood, sputum, urine, faeces, discharges from various places) and provides information on the sensitivity of bacteria to different antibiotics. Pathologists sometimes help to define and oversee certain hospital strategies and procedures, such as infection control.

Blood for tests may be obtained by venipuncture, the puncturing of a vein with a sharp needle, or sometimes from a finger prick if a small sample is required. The venipuncture may be performed by the doctor requesting the tests, a nurse or by staff attached to one of the laboratories. The specimen is usually taken from a prominent vein at the front of the forearm at or near the hollow of the elbow. Sometimes a cuff is applied further up the arm for a few seconds to help engorge the vein and improve blood flow. A prick may be felt as the needle first enters the skin but otherwise the procedure, when straightforward, is not usually particularly painful. Fear and anxiety are the main causes of distress associated with this procedure.

Blood is drawn into a syringe and then distributed into containers appropriate for the different laboratories and tests. Haematology tests mostly require whole blood. In order to obtain plasma the blood is spun in a tube at high speed in a centrifuge. The blood cells are forced to the bottom of the tube and the layer of plasma above can then be removed for testing. Special chemicals are added to the blood tubes to prevent clotting (unless serum is required).

Assessment of the meaning or importance of a test result requires, amongst other things, knowledge of what happens with that test in healthy people. Laboratories compile arbitrary limits above or below which a result might be suspected of having some significance. For instance, the lower and upper reference values for the total number of white blood cells in blood are usually given as four and eleven thousand million cells per litre respectively (in adults). Such reference ranges are based on the analysis of a large number of samples taken from the general population and are adjusted so that only a small proportion of subjects are above and below the limits. Often the limits are set to allow 95 per cent of people to fall between them. There is a tendency to avoid the term 'normal range' since by statistical definition a few healthy people are likely to fall outside it. On the other hand, if the limits are set too wide some results that do indicate disease or malfunction in particular individuals might be wrongly regarded as normal. A number of factors other than disease can affect laboratory tests and a good deal of caution is required when interpreting the results.

We shall now briefly consider the purposes of a few of the commonly requested laboratory tests.

Haemoglobin

Haemoglobin is the major constituent of red blood cells and it carries oxygen around the body. **Anaemia** is the condition in which there is an abnormally low level of circulating red cells and haemoglobin. Common causes are blood loss and iron deficiency (e.g. due to poor dietary intake of iron). Anaemia is relatively common in women of child bearing age because of blood losses during menstruation and childbirth. Another cause of anaemia is an increased rate of breakdown of the red cells; this is known as **haemolytic anaemia** (e.g. it occurs in sickle-cell disease). The definitive test for anaemia is the measurement of the concentration of haemoglobin in whole blood. The lower reference values for men and women are usually 130 and 115 grams of haemoglobin per litre of blood respectively (sometimes given as 13 and 11.5 g/100ml or decilitre).

White blood cell counts

The major white cells in blood are neutrophils (polymorphs) and lymphocytes. A few other types are present in smaller numbers. A **total white blood cell count** is the measurement of the total number of white cells in blood irrespective of their type. A **differential count** provides a breakdown of the total count in terms of the different types of white cell present. White cell counts may sometimes help to confirm the presence of infection or inflammation. The polymorph count often increases in bacterial infections and the lymphocyte count sometimes increases in viral infections. Very high white cell counts and abnormal looking white cells are usually present in untreated leukaemia.

Plasma urea and creatinine

As indicated earlier, urea is a simple molecule formed from excess nitrogen and is normally efficiently removed from the blood by the kidneys. The determination of the concentration of urea in plasma provides a simple assessment of kidney function. In renal failure the plasma urea concentration may be extremely high. Plasma creatinine concentrations provide an even better index of renal function. The muscles continually produce small amounts of creatinine, which is a substance of small molecular size not very dissimilar to urea. It passes into the bloodstream from which it is normally very efficiently removed by the kidneys and excreted into the urine. It is less prone than urea to the effects of the diet. By measuring creatinine in plasma and also in urine collected over a given time interval the **creatinine clearance** can be calculated. This parameter gives an approximate estimate of the glomerular filtration rate (see chapter two, page 40).

Plasma and urine glucose

Blood sugar is a common term which generally refers to the concentration of glucose in blood. In fact earlier tests did measure other sugars too, such as galactose, which also participates in metabolism but does not normally appear in significant amounts in plasma and urine (except in some very rare genetic disorders). Modern tests generally measure glucose specifically. The methods used in the laboratory provide accurate determinations over a wide range of concentrations. There are also simple methods involving chemically impregnated dipsticks that provide approximate estimates of glucose in urine (and some for blood too). These are used in general practice to assist in diagnosis and by patients with diabetes mellitus to help them monitor their treatment. Plasma glucose is excessively high in untreated or poorly controlled diabetes. Abnormally low levels are dangerous and are usually due to overtreatment with insulin.

Plasma bilirubin

The origin and fate of bilirubin was mentioned earlier on page 40. A number of conditions produce an increased concentration of bilirubin in plasma, which if high enough will be evident as jaundice. In general this is due either to an increased breakdown of red blood cells or to impaired handling and disposal of bilirubin in the liver or biliary system. Thus, typical causes of a raised plasma bilirubin are haemolytic anaemias such as sickle-cell disease and **haemolytic disease of the newborn** (due to incompatibility of mother's and baby's blood groups – e.g. antibodies made towards a Rhesus positive baby by a Rhesus negative mother), hepatitis, and obstructions in the tubes conducting the bile (e.g. a gall stone in the bile duct). However, about five per cent of the population have **Gilbert's syndrome**, a completely harmless familial condition characterised by a marginally high bilirubin level; slight jaundice sometimes occurs. This condition may occasionally cause confusion in diagnosis.

Plasma enzymes

Cell damage and abnormal cell proliferation cause enzymes to leak from the cells into plasma at a greater rate than they would normally. This forms the basis of some useful diagnostic tests. For instance, the plasma levels of a number of different enzymes are raised after a myocardial infarction. Hepatitis can cause very high enzyme levels. An elevation of the enzyme **acid phosphatase** in plasma may be an early sign of carcinoma of the prostate (raised levels may also occur after a rectal examination and after passing a large stool). The tests are not always that specific but certain combinations of plasma enzyme abnormalities sometimes point strongly to the involvement of a particular tissue or organ.

Electrolyte and acid-base determinations

In medicine the term **electrolytes** refers to certain ions in the body fluids, for instance sodium, potassium and chloride. **Acid-base** refers to components involved in the regulation of acidity, such as the hydrogen ion and bicarbonate (see chapter two, page 47). All of these constituents are normally tightly controlled by various feedback mechanisms. Diseases of the key organs involved in these processes may cause serious disturbances in electrolyte, water and acid-base balances. For instance, in advanced renal failure plasma potassium and blood hydrogen-ion concentrations may become dangerously high. Electrolyte and acid-base status require regular monitoring in such cases.

———— Electrocardiography ————

Electrocardiography is the technique of recording the electrical activity of the heart. The instrument used to do this is an **electrocardiograph** and the record it produces is an **electrocardiogram** (ECG). This test is used for the diagnosis of a number of cardiac disorders, including myocardial infarction. Electrocardiography is painless and **non-invasive**, that is it does not involve piercing the body with instruments. Compact portable machines are available. Hospital doctors and many general practitioners perform this very useful investigation.

Let us first review the physiological events in the normal heart. Special electrical conducting systems activate the heart muscles and cause them to contract. Normally, this activation proceeds in a set sequence and is carefully co-ordinated. The electrical field it incidentally generates around the heart can be detected by electrodes (simple metal plates) placed on the skin surface. The electrical activation precedes contraction of the muscle fibres. A typical recording of the voltage changes detected over the time period of the cardiac cycle is shown in figure 7.1. The main upward and downward deflections from the baseline on the standard ECG are designated by the letters P, Q, R, S, T. Two major signal complexes picked up at different times in the cardiac cycle are those due to activation of the muscles of the atria and ventricles. Activation of the

atria causes the **P wave** and activation of the ventricles causes the **QRS complex**. Figure 7.1 also indicates some of the
corresponding mechanical events in the heart. Note that the
QRS complex immediately precedes systole (contraction of the
ventricles and ejection of blood into the arterial system). The
T wave is the electrical signal corresponding to the start of
ventricular relaxation and is therefore closely followed by
diastole. You may at this point wish to consolidate your
understanding of the cardiac cycle by cross-referring to previous sections of relevance, such as that on auscultation in
chapter six, page 146.

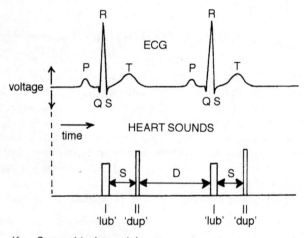

Key: S = ventricular systole
D = ventricular diastole

Figure 7.1 ECG and heart sounds from two consecutive heart beats

By placing the electrodes at different points on the body surface it is possible to focus the investigation on particular
anatomical aspects of the heart. For instance, an electrode
placed just beneath the left nipple will pick up strong signals
from the left ventricle, which tends to dominate and produces
the large R wave.

Electrodes (**leads**) are usually attached to the wrists and ankles (**limb leads**). Recordings are also taken at various places from the front to the left side of the chest wall (**chest leads**). A jelly is applied between electrode and skin to improve electrical conduction.

Typical ECG traces seen after a myocardial infarction are shown in figure 7.2. Note how the earliest changes may be seen within hours, often as a characteristic abnormal elevation of the baseline between S and T. Changes in this **S-T segment** also occur during attacks of angina pectoris, usually an abnormal depression rather than an abnormal elevation. Later and more permanent ECG changes after infarction may be an abnormally deep Q wave and abnormal T wave patterns. Analysis of the changes in the different leads may allow approximate identification of the site and extent of the infarct.

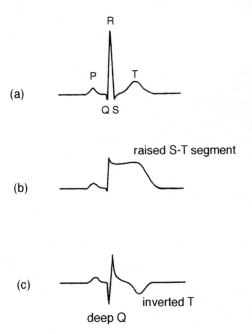

Figure 7.2 Typical ECG changes in a lead facing an area of myocardial infarction
(**a**) before infarction
(**b**) hours after infarction
(**c**) days after infarction

The ECG is useful in the diagnosis of many other cardiac disorders. Occasionally it is not helpful, even in some cases of myocardial infarction. ECG patterns normally vary slightly between healthy individuals, so small differences require careful interpretation.

Sometimes it is necessary to attach a small portable ECG unit with a tape recorder to the patient for several hours while they go about their normal activities. This may help to uncover sporadic cardiac events, such as occasional attacks of angina and arrhythmia.

Arrhythmias

We are now in a position to consider abnormal heart rhythms (**arrhythmias**) in a little more detail. Examination of the pulse and heart sounds provides some information about the rate and rhythm of the heart beat but electrocardiography is essential for the accurate diagnosis and management of arrhythmias. The ECG shows the electrical activity of the heart but it does not give any indication of the mechanical efficiency of the pump. Good electrical activity is no consolation in the absence of blood flow. Examination of pulse and blood pressure will provide mechanical information.

A special group of cells in the wall of the right atrium (the **sinus node**) normally paces the beating of the heart; it is the natural pacemaker. The autonomic nervous system influences its rate. The sinus initiates an electrical wave which first stimulates contraction of the atrial muscle and later the ventricles. The atrial and ventricular activities are co-ordinated by a special group of cells that conduct the electrical activating signal from the atrial muscle to the ventricular muscle. A delay in the transmission of this signal ensures that the atria beat first. The interval between the P wave and the QRS complex (the **P-R interval**) on the ECG is a measure of the conduction time between atrium and ventricle. Abnormal delays in conduction give rise to various forms of **heart block**. In complete heart block the ventricles beat completely independently of the atria, and at a much lower rate.

Abnormal heart rhythms may be **ventricular arrhythmias** or **supra-ventricular arrhythmias**. Ventricular arrhythmias arise from abnormal electrical activities in the muscles of the ventricles. They are mostly due to underlying heart disease, and are common after myocardial infarction. Two types are **ventricular tachycardia** and **ventricular fibrillation**. In ventricular tachycardia the ventricular rate may be as high as 200 beats per minute. Under such circumstances the pump is inefficient and the cardiac output is low. This may result in dizziness or even unconsciousness. Ventricular tachycardia is dangerous and must be treated promptly.

Ventricular fibrillation causes sudden death. The ventricles contract chaotically and there is no cardiac output, and therefore no pulse. Cardio-pulmonary resuscitation must be started immediately. A normal heart rhythm can often be restored by applying an appropriately controlled electric shock to the chest using a special piece of equipment known as a **defibrillator**. This is a routine procedure in coronary and intensive care units.

There are many different types of supra-ventricular arrhythmia, which may arise from aberrant signals in the atria or the specialised electrical conduction pathways. We shall just consider one, namely **atrial fibrillation**. In this condition the atrial muscle fibres beat chaotically at more than 400 beats per minute and the resultant erratic signals cause the ventricles to respond irregularly in time and strength. The ECG shows the absence of P waves. Blood normally flows freely from the atria to the ventricles during diastole. The atrial muscles normally contract towards the end of diastole and provide an extra boost to squeeze more blood into the ventricles. The absence of proper atrial contractions in atrial fibrillation does not necessarily seriously compromise cardiac output; atrial fibrillation is often symptomless. It may sometimes precipitate heart failure in people with pre-existing heart disease. The condition causes a chaotic heartbeat and a pulse which is irregular in rate and volume. There are many known causes of atrial fibrillation, including ischaemic heart disease, mitral stenosis, thyrotoxicosis and hypertension. Sometimes there is no apparent cause.

An important complication that can occasionally occur in atrial fibrillation, especially when there is co-existing mitral valve disease, is the formation of a blood clot in the left atrium. If the rhythm converts to normal in such circumstances there is a risk of embolism – the clot may then enter the systemic arterial system and lodge in a peripheral artery (e.g. a rarer cause of stroke).

X-rays

Several methods provide images of internal tissues and organs (**imaging**) without the need to open the body. One of the simplest and most widely used methods, which was also the earliest, involves the use of X-rays. Simple X-ray investigations can be extremely helpful in the diagnosis of many diseases. They are available in most hospitals and are relatively inexpensive.

X-rays are a form of radiation similar to radio waves, visible light, ultra-violet light and gamma rays (all forms of electromagnetic radiation). They differ only in their rate of vibration (frequency) and wavelength (which varies inversely with the frequency). Ordinary visible light has difficulty penetrating our tissues; X-rays and gamma rays pass through more readily. The higher the frequency of the radiation, the higher its energy. Gamma rays are emitted from some radioactive materials. They have extremely high frequencies, and therefore energies, require thick lead screens to block them and can damage living tissues. X-rays have frequencies that are lower than gamma rays but higher than ultra-violet rays. They penetrate the tissues of the body to a variable extent depending on the abundance of larger atoms (e.g. calcium, iron) which offer resistance. Excessive exposure to X-rays can be damaging. However, modern diagnostic X-ray techniques use small doses of radiation and can be considered safe when used prudently.

Although we cannot see them, X-rays can, like ordinary light, blacken photographic film (i.e. form negatives). Diagnostic X-rays are produced in a special type of lamp (X-ray tube). The rays shine through the patient onto the photographic plate. The calcium-rich bones block much of the radiation and appear as white images, whereas air, in the lungs for instance, offers little resistance and appears black. Soft tissues give intermediary shades. X-ray pictures are variously called radiographs, radiograms or just X-rays. Laser discs will probably eventually replace photographic plates as a means of storing the radiographic information.

X-ray pictures are taken with expensive equipment in purpose-designed facilities. The people operating the equipment and conducting the tests on a routine basis are the radiographers, who have a comprehensive scientific and technical training. They wear lead aprons to protect them from excessive exposure to radiation. Doctors specialising in this area of work are known as radiologists. They provide clinical interpretation of the pictures and advise on the use of this type of technique in diagnosis. They also undertake specialised X-ray investigations, sometimes with other clinical specialists.

X-ray investigations are used extensively in the diagnosis and management of disorders of the cardiovascular, respiratory and biliary systems, and alimentary and renal tracts. They are obviously important in the management of bone fractures.

The chest X-ray

The simple and relatively inexpensive chest X-ray is usually an essential part of the investigation of heart and lung disease. It complements the examination of the heart and may often pick up abnormalities in the lung when there are no signs present on physical examination. It may form part of a general medical screen. Mobile chest X-ray units have been very successful in screening susceptible populations for pulmonary tuberculosis.

Figure 7.3 illustrates a few of the features seen on a normal plain chest X-ray. Apart from the ribs (which are omitted for clarity), the most obvious radio-opaque area (i.e. pale area due to obstruction of the rays) is the large central mass due to the heart and its major vessels. It is not usually possible to distinguish the individual components within the cardiac shadow, but the edges and the shape and size of the silhouette can provide many useful diagnostic clues. The dark regions of the lungs contain a number of slightly radio-opaque markings due to various structures, particularly towards the centre.

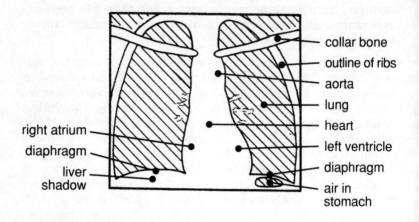

Figure 7.3 Some features of a chest X-ray

Abnormal shadows in the lung fields may be due to inflammation, fluid, tumour, enlarged lymph nodes, pulmonary oedema
and many other things. Sometimes pictures must be taken
from different directions and angles in order to accurately pinpoint the lesion anatomically and assess its characteristics in
greater detail.

Contrast radiography

The distinction between the different soft tissues, and clear
recognition of the outlines of some internal organs, can be difficult or imprecise using the straightforward X-ray method.
The outline of the heart is easily seen in the chest X-ray
because its shadow contrasts strongly against the blacker
image of the lungs. In some more specialised X-ray investigations the outlines of organs or body cavities are enhanced by
artificially improving their contrast against the surrounding
areas. This is usually done by introducing a radio-opaque
material (**contrast medium**) into the relevant part of the
body. These materials contain large atoms like barium or
iodine which can block X-rays even more effectively than bone.

The so-called **barium meal** allows the radiologist to study the
outline of the internal surface of the stomach and duodenum.

The contrast medium fills ulcer craters and flows over tumours, both lesions giving characteristic radiographic appearances. An enema containing barium is sometimes used in the investigation of large bowel disease.

Iodine-containing substances are used in the investigation of some biliary and renal diseases. One type, which is taken by mouth, is absorbed in the gut and then heavily excreted into the biliary system. X-rays of the abdomen taken at appropriate times after dosing can provide valuable information about gall bladder or bile duct disease. Another type of iodine-containing contrast medium is readily excreted by the kidneys after intravenous administration (injection into the systemic circulation via a vein). X-ray pictures are taken at intervals after the injection. Initially the contrast medium highlights the contour of the kidneys, thus providing information on their size and shape. Later it demarcates the urinary tract. The test provides useful information about renal tract structure and function.

Many other diagnostic X-ray tests utilise contrast media. Some are very specialised and involve the insertion of fine tubes into particular internal ducts or vessels. These invasive techniques require considerable expertise and often involve the collaboration of specialist clinician and radiologist. For example, **coronary angiography** involves selective release of contrast medium into the left and right coronary arteries. To do this a **catheter** (a long slender flexible tube through which fluid can pass) is inserted into a major artery, advanced through the aorta towards the heart and the tip positioned at the origin of the coronary artery (near the aortic valve). A rapid series of X-ray pictures is taken after release of small amounts of radio-opaque medium. Coronary angiography can reveal the extent and the precise location of atherosclerotic lesions. Such information is essential when considering the possibility of coronary artery surgery. A similar technique can be used to determine abnormalities in the arteries supplying the brain.

Scanners

A device that produces a good image of an internal organ or tissue is popularly known as a **scanner**. There are different types, with different advantages and disadvantages, but they all have in common the use of very sophisticated computer technology to assist image production. The main methods are **computed tomography** (**CT**; previously known as the **CAT** scan), **magnetic resonance imaging** (**MRI**) and **ultrasound**. They differ in the nature of the signal wave detected.

CT involves X-rays. It is particularly useful for obtaining images of abdominal organs. Multiple X-ray scans taken in rapid succession are analysed by computer image enhancing techniques to produce a picture of a slice through the body.

The physics of **MRI** is more complicated. Atoms subjected to a strong magnetic field and then probed by radio waves emit particular types of signals. The characteristics of these signals depend on the effects of other matter in the vicinity. Diagnostic MRI usually analyses such signals from the nuclei of hydrogen atoms. This technique provides excellent images of the brain, spinal cord and the organs in the pelvis. The instrument is very expensive and must be housed in a special facility. It generates an intense magnetic field. Objects attracted or affected by magnets (e.g. cardiac pacemakers) must be excluded from the vicinity of the machine.

Ultrasound techniques use high frequency sound waves which are outside the range of human hearing. The principle is similar to that of submarine sonar. The device emits ultrasonic signals and its detector receives the echos from various objects beneath the surface. The time delay gives a measure of the distance. Diagnostic ultrasound equipment ranges from the simple and inexpensive, which may not provide very good images but can sometimes usefully extend the scope of the physical examination, to the sophisticated high-tech versions used in cardiology. Ultrasound is particularly useful for examination of the female pelvis and for the detection of abnormalities in the fetus. It is also used in the investigation of the heart, kidney and liver. A special ultrasound device can determine the rate of blood flow in the heart chambers and in the great blood vessels arising from the heart.

Apart from the excellence of the images they produce, the above techniques have the great advantage of being basically non-invasive. CT and MRI are relatively expensive investigations and they are only available at special centres. Nevertheless, in some clinical situations they are the methods of choice and may then considerably cut the time and cost of investigation and be generally advantageous to the patient. Centres that regularly use advanced imaging techniques tend to devise policies and procedural guidelines to ensure the most efficient pathway to diagnosis in particular clinical circumstances, taking into account the advantages and disadvantages of the various methods, the patient's interests and the need to be cost-effective.

Endoscopy

Endoscopy is the examination of the inside of a hollow organ or cavity with a suitably narrow instrument (**endoscope**). It usually involves the insertion of the endoscope through the corresponding body orifice. By means of an optical system contained within the device the doctor can examine the interior of a tract or organ for abnormalities (e.g. ulcers, inflammation, tumours). Sometimes it is also possible to obtain a biopsy specimen during the procedure. There are several different types of endoscope, with names depicting their use. Some are flexible and some rigid. The **bronchoscope** is used for the trachea and larger bronchi and the **gastroscope** for the stomach and duodenum. The rectum and colon can be examined with the **sigmoidoscope** and **colonoscope**. A **cystoscope** is used to examine the bladder.

Sedatives may be given to reduce the patient's anxiety, and topical anaesthetic agents are applied to the sensitive surfaces as necessary before the procedure. Most endoscopy procedures cause some discomfort but they should not cause pain. Sometimes endoscopy is performed under general anaesthesia.

Particularly sophisticated endoscopic techniques are used in minimal access (keyhole) surgery (see chapter ten, page 223).

Simpler endoscopic examinations are often carried out as part of the physical examination. The **proctoscope** is a short tubular instrument for viewing the anal canal and the lower part of the rectum. It assists the investigation and treatment of **haemorrhoids** (piles, swollen veins in the region of the anus that tend to bleed or cause pain or discomfort). The vagina and cervix (the lower part of the womb that extends into the upper end of the vagina) are inspected by means of a **speculum**. This instrument separates the anterior and posterior walls of the vagina, which normally lie closely apposed, thus providing a better view and improved access (e.g. for taking a cervical smear).

8
PREVENTIVE MEDICINE

Introduction

In the nineteenth century the major cause of death in industrialised societies was infection. Subsequent public health measures and medical interventions dramatically reduced infectious disease. Today we still benefit from this. The average life expectancy is now 30 years longer than it was 100 years ago. Other diseases, appearing mainly in middle age or later life, contend as the major causes of death and suffering. Coronary artery disease, stroke and cancer now account for two-thirds of all deaths in the UK. There is good evidence that relatively simple preventive measures can reduce the risk of premature death from these conditions.

The purpose of preventive medicine is to reduce the risk of disease. One way of doing this is to reduce the risk from exposure to disease-causing agents (e.g. by removing sources of infection, by vaccination, by stopping smoking). A good example is the total eradication of smallpox following a worldwide vaccination campaign. Some of the diseases that plague us today are not caused by a single external agent but by the interaction of several factors, some external and some constitutional.

Another way of reducing risk is to detect disease at a much earlier stage, before it is evident clinically, to improve the chances of a cure (e.g. breast cancer) or at least to limit damage from the disease (e.g. hypertension, diabetes). Early detection of symptomless disease in the community involves the use of relatively simple tests that can be applied to large numbers of people (**screening tests**). A well known example is the cervical smear test for the early detection of cervical cancer (carcinoma of the cervix).

In the above examples the medical services clearly have important responsibilities. However, in some of the most important areas of preventive medicine in our society the ultimate responsibility for action rests with the individual. Personal health care and preventive medicine overlap. Keeping fit and preventing or reducing the likelihood of certain diseases depend very much on the way we live. Most of us could improve our fitness and health prospects considerably by adopting a healthier lifestyle. People often prefer to blame someone or something else rather than to do the obvious themselves, such as giving up smoking. The health of the individual, and sometimes those around them, may be put at risk through ignorance and attitude problems (e.g. spreading infection, unsafe practices in the home and at work). Education and training in health and safety matters is of crucial importance, and it should start at an early age.

A number of organisations provide advice on healthier living. Some represent the views of health professionals, some are state sponsored, some are commercially-oriented, some appear cranky. Many offer basically good advice, but the options can be confusing and sometimes conflicting. Incomplete scientific evidence on some issues, disagreements between experts, the real or imagined agendas of organisations, and media hype tend to breed dogma and scepticism. There is, however, no doubt that some relatively simple measures can substantially reduce the risk from a number of serious diseases. The primary health care teams can provide advice on preventive measures and healthier living; indeed they now have a mandate to do so. They will also conduct, or arrange and co-ordinate, specific screening tests and provide follow-up advice and treatment when necessary.

Social and economic factors are also important in the emergence of preventable disease. Those at the bottom of the socioeconomic ladder have a much higher incidence of heart disease and stroke. Infectious tuberculosis is becoming a major problem in the homeless populations of the UK. Social deprivation, family disruption, poverty, homelessness and unemployment can all adversely affect mental health, the motivation, the will and the means to improve lifestyle. Crowded and insanitary living conditions encourage the spread of infection. For some, cigarettes and alcohol may be the only comforts in a miserable and degrading life.

– Risk factors and disease prevention –

The risk factor was introduced in chapter three, page 54. It is a thing, a state or an action that increases the chances of contracting a disease. It may be a direct cause or it may help facilitate the activity of the causative agent, perhaps by allowing easier access or by enhancing the pathological process. For instance, measles can only occur after exposure to the measles virus but lack of immunity to the virus greatly increases the risk of contracting the disease. Several risk factors may operate in disease processes such as coronary atherosclerosis and cancer in which there may be an additive or cumulative effect, the more factors operating the greater the risk. Epidemiological research seeks associations between risk factors and disease. Modern scientific and statistical methods take into account the compounding effect of one factor upon another in order to determine the true risk attributable to each individual factor. This is not always easy. In some areas the evidence is still incomplete.

Preventive medicine aims to reduce the occurrence of a disease by modifying the factors that are known to increase the risk of contracting it. Many studies over many years have provided valuable information. There is now strong evidence that a few preventive measures, if adopted by the whole population, could substantially reduce the occurrence of many serious diseases and reduce the individual's chances of contracting them.

Sometimes vocal pressure groups crusade for changes because they believe that particular factors affect our health. Assisted by the media, they ensure that important issues are brought to our attention and are considered by those responsible for the national health. Authoritative professional bodies, and government departments, may occasionally appear slow or even reluctant to accept the need for such changes. This is rarely due to sloth. There are many considerations. All the available evidence must be examined, not just selected information. The validity of the data must be taken into account – not all research work is scientifically, technically and statistically sound. Opinions from leading experts and learned organisations must be gathered. Even when the evidence is convincing, the introduction of a recommendation or intervention on a national scale may not be straightforward. The individuals most at risk may not be identifiable in advance, so the preventive measure may need to be applied to the whole population. Those not at risk would gain little advantage; for them the risks of the measure may outweigh its benefits. The possible disadvantages and adverse effects of interventions and recommendations on the population as a whole must be considered.

Lifestyle risk factors are those that we inflict on ourselves and are generally under our control. They are of great importance and include smoking, unhealthy diets and lack of physical activity. Environmental risk factors may in addition require action by organisations, such as industry and government. Some risk factors require special detection methods and medical treatment (e.g. diabetes, hypertension).

—— Important lifestyle risk factors ——

There are many things that we can do to improve our health and lessen the risk of disease. Some of the major lifestyle risk factors are reviewed below. Doing something about them is often easier said than done. It may require considerable will power and some effort. And what exactly should we do? Valid scientific opinion can prove difficult to translate into clear and credible advice for the public at large. Helpful practical information on healthy eating, physical activity and many other health care topics is available from the Health Education Authority. Primary health care teams and the information units of local health authorities also provide advice and information.

Smoking

Smoking causes one-sixth of all deaths in the UK and US. It causes most of the deaths from lung cancer, chronic bronchitis and emphysema. It accounts for a quarter of the deaths from coronary heart disease and is a major factor in peripheral vascular disease. Smoking is an important risk factor for many other diseases too, including some other cancers. At present in the UK, smoking kills about 100,000 people every year. Had these people never smoked, they would probably have lived an average of at least ten years longer.

The longer a person smokes and the more smoke they inhale the greater the risk. Heavy cigarette smokers are about 30 times more likely to get lung cancer than life-time nonsmokers. After complete cessation of smoking the risk of lung cancer gradually diminishes over the next few years; the risk of coronary thrombosis decreases more rapidly.

The single most important disease prevention measure for smokers is to stop smoking. But giving up smoking is not easy for many people and they may need good advice and support to help them do it. Persuading young people not to start smoking is a major public health challenge.

Dietary factors

Nutrients, energy, foods and diets

We should first consider a few basic principles.

Nutrients are the individual substances that need to be present in food to ensure our continued life, health, growth and reproduction. The body normally extracts most of them very efficiently from the food we eat and utilises them in its metabolic processes. Nutrients may be grouped into carbohydrates (sugar-containing substances), fats, proteins, vitamins and minerals. Some nutrients are absolutely essential because we cannot make them from other materials (e.g. vitamin C, iron). Proteins in food generally contain all or most of the 20 amino acids found in human proteins, but their composition is very variable. Normally in adults eight particular amino acids are indispensable (methionine, phenylalanine, threonine, tryptophan, isoleucine, leucine, lysine, valine) and must be present in dietary protein in adequate amounts; the other twelve can be made in sufficient amounts by the body if necessary. Proteins of animal origin (e.g. those in milk, eggs, fish, meat) are generally richer in these essential amino acids than those of plant origin.

If our daily intake of an essential vitamin or mineral regularly falls below a certain minimum level we can become deficient in that substance. Initially this causes biochemical changes in the body, but eventually it may cause overt disease (e.g. vitamin C deficiency can cause scurvy). We differ in our average daily requirements. A number of authoritative bodies produce guidelines for the amounts of nutrients that we should consume to stay healthy. With the exception of food energy, these amounts are usually larger than the average individual requirements because they are meant to cover the requirements of most of the people most of the time. They are best known as RDAs (recommended daily amounts or allowances), although scientists sometimes use other terms. Food labels and packages often describe products in terms of these values. The nutrient intakes of most people in developed countries exceed their everyday needs (iron is an exception in some women). The body efficiently disposes of these substances when they are surplus to requirements. However, grossly excessive intakes of some nutrients (e.g. vitamins A and D) can lead to illness.

Fats and carbohydrates are the main fuels providing energy for the body. This energy drives the chemical processes and can be converted to heat (to maintain body temperature) or movement (muscular activity). The body carefully regulates the balance between energy input and energy output. The daily amounts of food energy that we require vary considerably and depend on factors such as our sex, age, body size, physical activity and individual metabolism. If we continually eat more energy-providing substances than we need the excess is stored as fat and we eventually become obese. Therefore, official recommendations for energy intakes do not include extra allowances but represent average requirements for particular groups of people.

The units used to measure energy in food tend to cause confusion. The best known unit is the Calorie (the large calorie). Unfortunately, this is not the same as the small calorie previously used in the physical sciences. The dietary Calorie is in fact equal to 1,000 calories (it is a kilocalorie or kcal). So you may see the energy (or calorific) content of fat given as nine Calories per gram or 9 kcal/gram. Typical average daily energy requirements for a man and woman might be say 2,600 and 2,000 kcal respectively. A man performing heavy manual work might require say 3,400 kcal per day. But remember, we all have our own individual requirements. In fit non-obese people energy intake closely matches the body's requirements.

We eat foods rather than individual nutrients. Foods such as bread, potatoes, beans, cereals, fish, meats, eggs, milks and cheeses contain carbohydrates, fats, proteins, vitamins and minerals but in very different amounts. Meats and fish are high in protein; bread and potatoes are high in carbohydrate. Some foods are deficient in particular vitamins and minerals. We need to eat a good variety of different types of food in order to supply the body with all the nutrients it requires. The combination of foods and drinks that we regularly consume constitutes our diet. A vegetarian diet can be very healthy providing it contains a suitable mixture of foods, and an adequate supply of iron and vitamin B_{12}.

The nutrient content of foods is usually determined by chemical analysis. The body may not receive these theoretical amounts. Some nutrients may be lost or damaged during the cooking or storage of food. Some may be chemically trapped in certain foods and may be less available to the body. The absorption of some nutrients is carefully controlled to prevent overload and toxicity (e.g. iron).

Not everything in the diet can be completely broken down and absorbed in the small intestine. This is particularly true of dietary fibre (roughage) which consists largely of indigestible complex carbohydrates. Dietary fibre comes mainly from cereals, vegetables and fruit. It adds bulk to the faeces and can be medically beneficial.

Nutritional disorders

Starvation and malnutrition (deficiency of essential nutrients) due to insufficient food and poor quality diets are still major problems in many parts of the world. Malnutrition is uncommon in developed countries but it can and does occur in certain vulnerable groups such as infirm elderly people who live alone, chronic alcohol abusers, and the urban poor. Nutritional deficiency states are occasionally caused by illness. In some diseases affecting the alimentary system food may be poorly digested or the nutrients poorly absorbed (e.g. cystic fibrosis, coeliac disease). Extensive tissue regeneration following injury or disease increases the body's requirements for nutrients. Particular attention should be given to the diet during illness and convalescence. Malnutrition reduces the ability of the body to combat infections.

The major nutritional disorders in developed countries are due mainly to overeating high energy foods (leading to obesity) or eating particular types of foods in undesirable amounts.

Diet and heart disease

Many factors influence the development of coronary atherosclerosis and subsequent angina or myocardial infarction – some were mentioned in chapter three, pages 57-9. A high plasma cholesterol level is one of the risk factors. The diet influences plasma cholesterol. The relationship between diet, cholesterol and fat metabolism and coronary disease, and the underlying mechanisms, are very complicated and not fully understood. But much is known and certain generalisations can be made. The amount of saturated fat (**saturates**) in the diet appears to be the most important dietary factor influencing plasma cholesterol levels. High levels of saturates in the diet are associated with higher cholesterol levels and with a higher risk of coronary artery disease. Furthermore, many studies have shown that a reduction in dietary saturates can reduce the risk of coronary artery disease.

What exactly are saturates? The fat in our food and in our bodies consists mainly of **triglycerides**. Triglycerides are formed when the simple molecule **glycerol** combines chemically with three **fatty acid** molecules. This is illustrated in figure 8.1. In its pure form glycerol is a sweet syrupy liquid (also called glycerin). The -O-H groups attached to the carbon atoms in the glycerol molecule are known chemically as alcohol groups (not to be confused with alcohol in wine, beer, etc.).

TWO COMMON FATTY ACIDS

palmitic acid

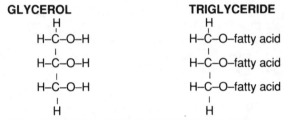

oleic acid

GLYCEROL

TRIGLYCERIDE

CIS AND TRANS FORMS OF DOUBLE BOND

cis

trans

Figure 8.1   Fatty acids, glycerol and triglyceride

They are different from and do not form ions like the hydroxyl groups in alkalis (see chapter two, page 47). The *fatty* part of a fatty acid molecule consists of a long chain of carbon atoms surrounded by hydrogen atoms. At one end there is a small group of atoms (carboxyl group; -CO.OH) which confers acidic properties to the molecule. The H in the carboxyl group can break away to form a hydrogen ion (H^+). The carboxyl groups on the fatty acids react with the alcohol groups on glycerol to form triglyceride (enzymes facilitate the reaction). The acid groups disappear. The triglycerides are very fatty and insoluble in water. There are different types of fatty acid molecule, and triglycerides usually contain a mixture. They differ in the number of carbon atoms in the chain and in the way some of the carbon atoms are linked together. In **saturated fatty**

acids there are only single bonds linking the carbon atoms together. One of the saturates capable of raising plasma cholesterol levels is called **palmitic acid**, it has 16 carbon atoms in its chain (figure 8.1). **Unsaturated fatty acids** (**unsaturates**) have double bonds between particular carbon atoms in the chain; the molecule is therefore less saturated with hydrogen atoms. Those with just one double bond are called **monounsaturates** (e.g. oleic acid, a component of olive oil) and those with more than one are called **polyunsaturated fatty acids**. A final point is that the double bond can produce two different types of spatial kink in the carbon chain, thus giving rise to the so-called cis and trans fatty acids (figure 8.1, page 175). Natural foods, especially vegetables, contain mainly cis forms. The proportion of trans fatty acids is higher in margarines and some spreads, and in deep-fried foods. The role of trans fatty acids in human disease is uncertain and is still the subject of debate and research.

Polyunsaturated fatty acids (**PUFAs**), in relatively large amounts, can actually lower plasma cholesterol. Some PUFAs are essential nutrients, but only small amounts are needed. The average British diet is not rich in PUFAs but generally contains the essential requirements. There is some concern that high levels of these substances in the diet could lead to other problems, but the evidence is not yet conclusive. The amount of cholesterol in the diet (e.g. from eggs) also influences plasma cholesterol but the relationship is not straightforward. Plasma cholesterol comes from the diet and from the liver, which makes cholesterol. When dietary cholesterol increases, the production of cholesterol in the liver decreases. Nevertheless, diets high in cholesterol tend to increase plasma cholesterol concentrations. The effect differs between individuals and there are genetic influences. The composition of the diet can also affect the activities of the blood clotting mechanisms and this may be one of the factors influencing the onset of coronary thrombosis.

Diet is important in the development of atherosclerosis and coronary artery disease. However, it is not the only factor. Furthermore, the fact that changes in the average national diet can reduce the overall occurrence of heart disease in the population does not provide guarantees for the individual.

Diet and cancer

There is compelling evidence that the composition of the diet influences the risk of developing certain cancers (e.g. carcinoma of the stomach, large bowel or breast). The nature of the food substances involved and their mechanisms of action are not clear. Nevertheless, and fortunately, there are good reasons to believe that the type of diet that might reduce the risk of cancer is generally compatible with that now recommended for the prevention of heart disease.

Potential carcinogens are sometimes found in food. They may be chemicals occurring naturally in particular foods, substances formed by high-temperature cooking methods, or contaminants introduced incidentally or accidentally during farming or storage. The role of these substances in the genesis of cancer in developed countries is uncertain and still under investigation.

The healthy diet

A diet regularly over-rich in saturates and poor in fruits and vegetables increases the risk of atherosclerosis and cancer. Vegetarians have a lower incidence of both diseases, even when non-dietary lifestyle differences are taken into account. The main sources of saturates are full-fat dairy products, lards and meat products.

At present 40 per cent of the energy (kcals) in the average British diet comes from fats (all fats, including oils) and 45 per cent from carbohydrates. Saturates currently account for about 15 per cent of the dietary energy. Recent recommendations are that saturates should provide no more than 10 per cent of the energy, and that total fat and carbohydrate should provide about 35 per cent and 50 per cent respectively. The remaining 15 per cent of energy is due mainly to protein and would remain unchanged. Alcohol is also an energy-providing fuel but by convention it is not included in the so-called dietary energy. Nevertheless, in many men who drink, alcohol commonly accounts for nearly a tenth of their total energy intake.

It has been suggested that the average vegetable, fruit, potato and bread consumption in the UK should be increased to compensate for the proposed reduction in energy from saturates. This would provide additional digestible complex carbohydrates like starch (an energy source) and additional dietary fibre (less digestible carbohydrates); both are thought to be beneficial. Adjustments in the diets of individuals obviously need to take into account the present composition of their diet and any special requirements. An adequate energy intake is vital, but not too much. All essential nutrients must be present in the diet in adequate amounts. Many vegetarians are already eating a healthy diet. Most people could adopt a healthier diet without too much difficulty and still enjoy eating; it is not necessary to become a vegetarian. Lean meats, poultry and fish, properly cooked, and in prudent amounts, are good foods. The average daily intake over a period (e.g. week) is the important criterion. The usual day-to-day variations are less important as the body can cope with this.

Overweight and obesity

Obesity is damaging to health. It increases the risk of developing cardiovascular disease, gall bladder disease, diabetes (type 2), osteoarthritis of the knees and hips, and even some cancers. The accumulation of fat around the middle of the body (abdomen and waist) is more strongly associated with cardiovascular disease than obesity affecting mainly the lower part of the body (hips and thighs). Prevention of overweight and obesity is important. Once established, obesity is difficult to treat – the existence of a vast and lucrative slimming industry is testimony to this.

Fatness is not easy to measure directly. However, a very useful and easily calculated guide applicable to most people is the Body Mass Index (BMI). This is the weight in kilograms (M, i.e. mass) divided by the square of the height in metres.

$$(BMI = M/H^2)$$

The desirable BMI is 20 to 25. A BMI of 25 to 30 indicates overweight (mild obesity) and a BMI of over 30 indicates obesity. A very muscular man can have a BMI of over 25 without being fat.

Obesity occurs when the energy intake chronically exceeds energy expenditure. A high fat diet, alcohol consumption and physical inactivity contribute to the development of obesity. The dietary recommendations mentioned in the preceding section together with adequate regular physical exercise should help prevent a person becoming overweight.

Established overweight and obesity is best treated with a combination of a suitable slimming diet and regular exercise. Individuals have different problems and requirements; professional advice may be required. Dieting *is* hard, but with persistence weight can be lost. Apart from the lower calorie content, the typical slimming diet is low in fat and alcohol. But it must contain adequate amounts of protein and essential vitamins and minerals. Crash dieting with a very low food energy intake is dangerous and should only be done under medical supervision.

Lack of exercise

About three-quarters of the UK population take too little exercise. Physical inactivity increases the risk of coronary artery disease and obesity. It may also be one of the factors that contribute to **osteoporosis**, a condition in which the bones lose substance and become weaker (see page 193).

Regular but moderate aerobic exercise taken throughout life is probably the most beneficial. Nevertheless, a suitable exercise program started at any age can be medically beneficial. Aerobic exercise involves working a reasonably large amount of muscle in order to increase the activities of the cardiovascular and respiratory systems (i.e. it needs to cause an increase in heart rate). Examples of aerobic exercise are walking (at a reasonable pace), jogging, skipping, running, dancing, cycling, many ball games and other active sports. A typical exercise session might last 20 to 30 minutes (perhaps an hour if walking), preferably at least three or four times a week. Strenuous exercise can sometimes cause problems, especially in the unfit and those unaccustomed to it. Exercise programmes should be tailored to individual needs; most people require advice. A preliminary medical assessment is advisable for those with pre-existing medical conditions and for middle-aged and elderly people before they embark on a physical fitness programme.

Alcohol

The problem of alcohol misuse and dependence was introduced in chapter five, page 132.

The chemical name for the type of alcohol that we consume in beers, spirits, wines etc. is ethanol (or ethyl alcohol). Its molecular structure was shown in figure 2.1, page 7. Ethanol is just one of several different chemicals which chemists call alcohols; they have in common the presence of an -O-H (alcohol) group. However, from here onwards we shall just refer to ethanol by its common name, alcohol. Alcohol consumption is conveniently measured in terms of units. One unit is ten millilitres of pure alcohol, which equates approximately to a half pint of ordinary strength beer or to a single (English – 25ml) measure of spirit. A small glass of wine (125ml) is often quoted as one unit, but this applies to wines containing eight per cent alcohol by volume; many contain around eleven per cent.

Chronic excessive alcohol consumption can cause disease in almost any organ or tissue. Obesity and hypertension may occur early on, thereby increasing the risk of cardiovascular disease, including stroke. Other serious consequences include brain degeneration (e.g. dementia), cancer of the gullet, damage to the heart muscle (cardiomyopathy), pancreatitis and liver disease. Initially the liver becomes fatty; this may reverse if drinking ceases. Hepatitis sometimes occurs. **Cirrhosis** of the liver may develop after a few years of excessive alcohol consumption.

Cirrhosis is characterised by widespread cellular damage, chronic inflammation and scarring in the liver. The loss of functioning liver cells results in underproduction of essential substances, such as blood clotting proteins, and an inability to remove toxic substances (which can sometimes lead to coma). Cirrhosis also damages the blood vessels in the liver thereby causing an abnormally high pressure in the portal venous system (see chapter two, page 39). This pressure transmits to the veins of the oesophagus and stomach, which may occasionally rupture and produce large haemorrhages into the alimentary canal.

So, what constitutes unsafe drinking from the medical viewpoint? The low-risk average daily consumption is considered to be no more than three units for men and two units for women. The higher the consumption above this level the greater the risk of disease, especially when the average daily consumption regularly exceeds about five units in men and three and a half units in women. Ironically, at low levels of consumption (e.g. less than two units) alcohol appears to be slightly protective against coronary artery disease. However, in view of the many problems associated with alcohol, including dependence, even light consumption cannot be recommended as a public health measure.

Even in small amounts, alcohol can impair performance and judgment. People differ in the way they handle and react to this drug. It should be avoided altogether before driving or performing potentially dangerous activities. The UK legal limit for blood alcohol when driving is 80mg/100ml (under review at the time of writing). But lower concentrations can cause mental impairment, especially in those who drink infrequently or who are also taking certain medications.

Alcohol spreads throughout and is diluted in all the water of the body. Women should in general drink less alcohol than men. This is because on average they have a smaller total body water volume and therefore get higher concentrations when drinking the same amount as men. Alcohol is absorbed in the stomach and intestine, and blood levels may rise quickly when concentrated alcoholic drinks are taken on an empty stomach; levels may reach a peak in half-an-hour. The presence of food in the stomach slows absorption. The liver is the main organ responsible for removing alcohol from the body, but it does this slowly, typically at about one unit per hour. Therefore high blood alcohol levels may still be present in the morning after an evening binge and may still be dangerous. The elimination of alcohol is often impaired in people who have, or have had, liver disease.

Other risks

There are many potential hazards around us. Some are avoidable and people need to be aware of them. Education and training are important in reducing many of these risks. Here we shall just consider a few.

Infection

The relatively low level of serious infections in developed countries does not just occur by chance. It is due to all the efforts made in the past and the procedures and practices in current use. It is a delicate balance. Some of the factors involved were discussed in chapter three. We can all make some contribution to keeping infection down. The most obvious way is to reduce the risk of exposure. This involves avoiding or removing the source of infection and/or preventing its spread. Sometimes this is impracticable. Many people travel in crowded buses and trains and are constantly exposed to airborne germs from coughs and sneezes. Fortunately, the diseases involved are usually minor upper respiratory tract infections, such as the common cold. We obviously have a responsibility not to knowingly infect other people. In practice it is sometimes difficult for people to stay away from work because of a mild cold. But they certainly should do so if they have a more serious infectious illness such as influenza, for the sake of others as well as themselves.

The risk of contracting a sexually transmitted disease (STD) can be reduced by limiting casual sex and the number of different partners, and by using a condom. The risk of developing serious illness from diseases such as gonorrhoea and syphilis can be reduced considerably if advice is sought early on. Confidential advice, a sympathetic attitude and specialist investigation and treatment for STD, without the need to go first to the general practitioner, are available in the genito-urinary medicine clinics (GUMs; previously called 'special clinics'), which are to be found in many large general hospitals and are available free as a walk-in service to all in the UK. These clinics play an important role in controlling the spread of STD.

Food poisoning due to bacterial infection causes illness in thousands of people in the UK every year; fortunately there are only a few fatalities. Hygiene and good practices in the home and in catering and food manufacturing and retailing establishments can greatly reduce the risk of food poisoning. This requires clean water supplies, good facilities, adequate training and in some cases regulation, inspection and enforcement. Personal hygiene is important in preventing the spread of infection in food. For instance, hands should be washed after handling raw food, touching the face and hair, handling money, smoking, blowing the nose and, of course, going to the toilet. There are always a few germs around and the best way to limit their multiplication is to carefully regulate the temperature and duration of food storage and cooking. Bacteria multiply rapidly in food at room and body temperatures. To prevent bacterial growth during temporary storage (e.g. a few hours) food needs to be kept sufficiently cold (less than 5°C) or hot (more than 63°C). Inadequate thawing of frozen poultry has often resulted in undercooking and consequent food poisoning. Care must also be taken not to allow raw food to contaminate cooked food (e.g. raw food should not be stored above cooked food in a refrigerator).

Many people do not take adequate precautions when travelling abroad to places where serious infections are known to occur. Medical advice should be sought. The risk of contracting malaria can be reduced by taking antimalarial drugs a week before going abroad, during the visit and for four weeks after returning. In recent years the malarial parasite has in many parts of the world become more resistant to antimalarial drugs; it is therefore very important that the right drugs are taken. Another way to decrease the risk of infection is to increase the body's resistance to it by immunisation (see page 186).

Unintended injury

Accidents, that is unintended injuries, account for about two per cent of all deaths in the UK. They are the biggest single cause of death in children and young adults, and for every death there are hundreds of non-fatal injuries, many leading to serious disability. Injury is therefore one of the most important causes of loss of useful years of life and work. Nevertheless, the death rate from accidents in the UK is one of lowest, and it is steadily falling. Alcohol is an important factor in accidents and intentional violence.

Road traffic accidents (RTAs) are the commonest cause of accidental death in young adults, mainly as drivers or passengers. Important factors contributing to RTAs are alcohol and speed. Factors determining severity of injury are speed and personal and vehicle safety features. Failure of many cyclists and horseriders to wear protective headgear causes an unnecessary number of serious head injuries. When the elderly are involved in RTAs they are more likely to be pedestrians; confusion and poor sight and hearing probably contribute. Legislation on drink-driving, personal and vehicle safety measures and speed limits has helped to reduce RTAs, but more needs to be done.

Falls are a major cause of injury in the elderly, and especially of fractured hips in elderly women. Many falls are caused by deteriorating function (e.g. poor vision, weakness, poor co-ordination, dizziness due to blood flow changes) and external hazards (e.g. things on the floor or pavement causing trips and slips). Prescribed drugs such as sleeping pills, antidepressants and tranquillisers are also important causes of falls in the elderly.

Ultraviolet radiation

Excessive exposure to the ultraviolet (UV) radiation in sunlight can seriously damage the skin and cause skin cancer. Those most at risk are fair-skinned people, especially those who do not tan and tend to burn easily in the sun. People with dark skins are protected by the pigment and are less susceptible. Repeated sun bathing accelerates the aging process in the skin, which becomes prematurely thin and wrinkled. The most serious consequence of overexposure is skin cancer, which occurs most frequently in Australia but is increasing in the UK and US. Genetic factors are thought to be important in skin cancer as well as excessive exposure to sunlight.

There are different forms of skin cancer. The commonest types account for 10 per cent of all cancers, but fortunately the cure rate is high and death from these tumours is uncommon. They are caused by many years of exposure to the sun and not surprisingly occur mainly on the most exposed parts of the body (e.g. the face).

The malignant melanoma (a darkly pigmented tumour) is a rarer form of skin cancer, but it is more dangerous and is associated with a much higher death rate. The prognosis can be good if the tumour is detected and properly removed at an early stage. Initially many melanomas appear as irregular pigmented patches or plaques. About a third arise in a pre-existing mole, but the vast majority of benign moles do not become malignant. Excessive exposure to sunlight is an important cause of malignant melanoma.

Prevention of skin cancer obviously involves avoiding excessive exposure to sunlight. Great care should be taken not to allow the skin to get burnt, and this applies to children too. Protective sunscreen products can be applied to exposed skin to filter out the harmful rays. Different skin types need different strengths of sunscreen. Most pharmacies can offer advice. The Australian public health message is 'SLIP, SLAP, SLOP – slip on a shirt, slap on a hat, slop on the sunscreen'.

Early detection of tumours is important. The skin is prone to develop many small lumps, bumps and pigmented areas. Most are completely harmless. It is not always easy to decide whether a particular skin lesion is likely to be troublesome. Medical advice should be sought when a lump continues to grow, itches, bleeds or ulcerates, when a new mole appears, or when changes occur in an existing mole. A doctor might suspect malignant melanoma if the lesion shows a few of the following features: itching, increasing in size, asymmetry, irregular border, irregular surface, irregularity or variety of colour (e.g. black, browns, blues, reds, white), inflammation, bleeding or crusting.

Asbestos

Asbestos is a fibrous mineral which has been widely used in industry, especially for insulating buildings and ships. Inhalation of asbestos dust can cause severe lung disease which may not become fully apparent until many years later.

A combination of smoking and exposure to asbestos greatly increases the risk of carcinoma of the lung. One unusual and relatively uncommon form of cancer is particularly associated with previous, and sometimes trivial, exposure to asbestos dust – this is **mesothelioma**, a highly malignant tumour of the pleura (and sometimes the peritoneum). Although industry has in general taken measures to eliminate the use of and reduce exposure to asbestos the number of people dying from mesothelioma may continue to rise for some years because of the large number of people previously exposed. The disease may not appear until some 15 to 40 years after exposure, but if it does it is invariably fatal within a year. Other factors are involved because the majority of people who have been exposed to asbestos dust have not developed the disease.

Many buildings still contain asbestos. Therefore building workers, plumbers and electricians, for instance, still need to be particularly vigilant and take necessary precautions.

Immunisation

A natural infection induces a defensive response in the immune system. Afterwards, the lymphocytes retain a memory of the antigens of the organism responsible and are then able to react more vigorously and therefore provide better immune protection to any future infection by the same organism (see chapter three, page 87). Immunisation is an artificial means of providing such immune protection without the need to suffer the risks and ravages of the natural infection. There are two types of immunisation, passive and active.

Passive immunisation involves the administration of immunoglobulins (antibodies) with specific activity against the offending organism or toxin. It does not stimulate the body to produce antibodies against the disease. This method is used when immediate protection is required for possible imminent life-threatening infection or toxicity (e.g. after a bite from a rabid dog). For many years the protective immunoglobulins were administered in the form of a **serum** (an **antiserum**). Nowadays more purified preparations are often available. The administered immunoglobulins are gradually degraded by the body and protection only lasts for a few weeks, but this may be sufficient to help prevent the disease.

Active immunisation (vaccination) involves the administration of a vaccine containing the antigenic material of the organism. This is the usual type of immunisation and it can provide long-lasting protection. Most vaccines are injected into a tissue. The polio vaccine used in children is given by mouth. Vaccines may contain live organisms (e.g. measles, mumps, rubella and oral polio vaccines), killed organisms (e.g. whooping cough vaccine), inactivated bacterial toxin (e.g. tetanus vaccine) or relatively pure antigen (e.g. some hepatitis B vaccines). The organisms or other antigenic materials present in vaccines are modified in order to produce the protective immune response without actually causing the disease. Repeat vaccinations (booster doses) are often necessary to sustain high levels of immunity. Live vaccines tend to provide the best immune protection; the organisms are gradually destroyed by the body's defence systems. Newer technologies are producing vaccines that are more purified and more tailored with the prospect of greater efficacy and fewer problems.

In the UK, parents are advised to have their children immunised against whooping cough (pertussis), diphtheria, tetanus, measles, mumps, rubella, poliomyelitis, tuberculosis and, recently, Haemophilus influenzae type B infection (Hib; an important cause of meningitis in young children, but not the only cause). People who travel abroad or who are at particular risk (e.g. because of their job) can be immunised against a variety of infections, such as typhoid, tetanus, polio, plague, rabies, hepatitis, meningococcal meningitis and yellow fever. Influenza vaccination can provide valuable protection for people at special risk from the infection, such as those with chronic lung disease. Travellers should obtain up-to-date advice on the recommended vaccination schedules for the countries they intend to visit.

Immunisation is an extremely effective method of preventing infection. Very occasionally the immune response may not be sufficient to completely prevent infection, but in such cases the disease is often less severe than it would have been without prior vaccination. The potential benefit from an officially recommended vaccination, in terms of reduced risk of damage from infection, usually far outweighs the risk of possible harmful effects from the vaccine itself.

For the vast majority of the population immunisation is an extremely safe procedure. A few individuals are more prone to harm from the vaccine. Live vaccines are avoided in pregnant women and patients with depressed immune function (e.g. those on immunosuppressive drugs after organ transplantation). Vaccination is usually avoided in people who are unwell, have a fever, have had previous bad reactions to the vaccine or are known to be allergic to components in the vaccine (e.g. egg protein in flu vaccines). Vaccination may produce mild side effects such as a slight fever, or local inflammation or a small lump at the injection site. A small proportion of infants are prone to convulsions when they are feverish (fever fits). This may also occur very occasionally after vaccination. Different vaccines have different precautions to be observed and instructions to be followed, and may have their own peculiar side effects. Such information is readily available to the public from clinics and health education organisations. Medical advice should always be sought if there are concerns about suitability for immunisation or if side effects occur.

Public concern over reports of brain damage apparently associated with pertussis (whooping cough) vaccination in children led to a fall in the number of children being immunised in the UK. As a result the infection has become more common again and there has been an increase in death and serious damage from the disease. Consensus medical opinion is that pertussis vaccination is most unlikely to cause brain damage. The potential benefits of immunisation against pertussis greatly outweigh any risks from the vaccine itself.

In the case of infectious organisms that reside and breed only in man (e.g. measles), immunisation of most of the susceptible population (mass vaccination) not only protects those vaccinated but can also reduce the spread and prevalence of the disease in the whole population. In theory co-ordinated mass vaccination could completely eradicate such organisms and the diseases they cause. This has actually been achieved in the case of smallpox. The World Health Organisation and many national immunisation campaigns hope to achieve this for some other diseases. For very infectious diseases this is only possible when almost all of the susceptible population agree to be vaccinated. When a disease has been totally eradicated there is of course no further need for vaccination against it. But when low rates of infection still occur in partially immunised populations, the usual case, continuation of vaccination is important. In such circumstances a decrease in vaccination produces a lower level of immunity in the population and the risk of subsequent epidemics of the infection. Furthermore, non-immune adults sometimes suffer more serious effects when they acquire some of the infections traditionally more common in children. Worries about epidemics of whooping cough, measles and other infectious diseases have led to a drive to increase the level of vaccination in children in the UK.

Early detection of disease

Screening tests

Many procedures and tests are capable of detecting symptomless disease but this does not necessarily mean that they are useful or practicable for screening large numbers of people. Some are useful for diagnosis when used in combination with other findings, but on their own they may be too nonspecific or unreliable. Many factors need to be taken into account before embarking on a mass screening programme; these may concern the disease itself, the population to be screened, the test, the consequences and follow-up of positive results, organisation, and whether the benefits justify the use of limited health service resources.

Earlier diagnosis needs to offer some advantage to the patient, such as the prospect of a better prognosis through earlier treatment. For some diseases this is not the case, or a treatment may not be available at all. When possible, screening tests are first studied as a research project using a limited population. This helps to determine the reliability of the test in practice, whether the disease really can be detected substantially earlier or an increased risk predicted more reliably than with existing procedures, and whether earlier treatment resulting from this really does improve the prognosis.

Tests are rarely 100 per cent reliable and accurate. The performance of a screening test can often be adjusted to make it more or less capable of detecting the abnormal. At first sight, one might think that such tests should never be allowed to miss an abnormal finding. If this were the case, the test would produce no **false negative** results (results indicating absence of disease when disease is actually present) but it would then also be very likely to produce an unacceptably high number of **false positive** results (results indicating presence of the disease when it is actually absent). All positive results must be further investigated to confirm the presence or absence of the disease. A careful balance must be struck between the levels of false negatives and false positives, for the sake of those being screened and in order to make the screening programme practicable and economically viable.

There are many other considerations in the successful operation of population screening. Adequate resources, training, organisation, administration and quality control, good management, and effective and efficient follow-up of positive results are all essential. In the past some of these elements have been deficient in some screening programmes (e.g. cervical cancer), which has on occasions led to unacceptable situations. Fortunately, there have now been improvements.

The following sections briefly review some of the screening tests currently used for the early detection or prediction of disease.

Hypertension

Hypertension is often symptomless for many years before it eventually causes serious disease. Early treatment reduces the risk of stroke. The primary health care teams in the UK are contracted to check the blood pressure of all adults on their registers at least every five years.

Plasma cholesterol

There is an association between plasma cholesterol and the risk of developing coronary heart disease. The lowering of high plasma cholesterol levels by diet or drug treatment is associated with a reduction in this risk. When screening a population, plasma cholesterol measurements will, for several reasons, inevitably produce a large number of false positive and false negative results in terms of predicting the outcome for individuals. A very high cholesterol level does carry a much higher risk. In such cases there may already be a family history of early heart disease. A high plasma cholesterol level is only one of several important risk factors for coronary artery disease, and it is less influential in the absence of the other risk factors. Also, a low plasma cholesterol level does not exclude the possibility of developing the disease. Furthermore, individuals can opt for the healthier diet and lifestyle without the need for such measurements. For these, and other reasons, there is some controversy over the advantages and practicality of screening everyone's plasma cholesterol.

The present medical consensus in the UK is that plasma cholesterol should be measured in people who also have other identifiable risk factors (e.g. smoking, obesity, hypertension, diabetes, etc.) and/or a family history of premature death from coronary heart disease (e.g. before 50 years in men, before 55 in women). Nevertheless, cholesterol self-screening tests are readily available to the public (e.g. from pharmacies) and individuals can have the test done privately if they so wish. Medical advice and counselling is required when a screening test gives a high value. Also, the results from simple, and possibly not very accurate, screening tests often require confirmation using professionally acceptable procedures, both in terms of blood sampling and laboratory methods.

Breast cancer

The earlier detection of breast cancer that is now possible using special X-ray techniques (mammography) allows earlier treatment and the prospect of a lower death rate from breast cancer in women over 50 years. General practitioners in the UK are now required to invite all women in the age range 50 to 64 to attend special mammography screening centres every three years. The test is less effective in premenopausal women. As with many screening tests there will be some true positive results (breast cancer present), a larger number of false positives and technical problems making the interpretation of some results difficult. This means that a proportion of patients will be asked to attend for additional tests. Only a small proportion of these follow-up patients will actually have breast cancer.

Regular breast self-examination (BSE) has been advocated as a means of detecting palpable tumours as early as possible. It usually involves initial instruction in technique and, traditionally, regular monthly self-examination. In premenopausal women this is best done just after the period has finished. Monthly BSE has apparently not been as beneficial as was originally hoped and some doctors now advocate a less regimented approach with an emphasis on 'breast awareness'. Early detection and treatment are key factors in prognosis. Unfortunately, many women who do detect lumps in their breasts delay seeking medical advice.

Cervical cancer

Cervical cancer is not very common but it accounts for more than 2,000 deaths in women every year, and the prevalence of the disease is expected to increase. Factors which may predispose women to cervical cancer include smoking and infection with a virus (**human papilloma virus, HPV**), the spread of which might be reduced by more widespread use of the condom. Fortunately, invasive carcinoma of the cervix is preceded by premalignant or noninvasive stages in which the affected cells may be discretely localised for some time in a small area of cervix. These early lesions can be removed by simple techniques which provide a complete cure. Simple cervical screening techniques can detect cervical cancer at the earliest and most treatable stages. Evidence suggests that more than 80 per cent of deaths from this disease might be prevented by effective five-yearly screening of all women over the age of 20. Three-yearly screening is slightly better, but more frequent screening appears to offer little further advantage.

In the UK, at least five-yearly (and often 3-yearly) cervical screening is now available via the general practitioner to all women aged 20 to 64. Past experience suggests that many women in inner city areas, some of whom are more prone to the disease, are less likely to attend for screening and may need more encouragement.

Other screening activities

There are a number of other screening tests available for the early detection of disease or disease risk. Newborn babies are routinely tested for the presence of congenital hypothyroidism and phenylketonuria (see chapter four, page 113). Untreated, both of these disorders can lead to severe mental retardation. Treatment is available and it is effective if started as soon as possible after birth. In some areas infants are screened for sickle-cell disease. Newborn babies are routinely examined for physical abnormalities. Children are also screened for other conditions, such as impaired hearing.

There are many tests for the detection of fetal abnormalities during pregnancy. Some are very specialised and are only used in certain situations – for instance, the prenatal (antenatal) diagnosis of rare severe genetic disorders where there is already a relevant family history of the disease. In such circumstances the detection of the abnormality early in pregnancy provides an opportunity for the parents to consider the possibility of terminating the pregnancy, should they so wish. More common antenatal screens are the use of ultrasound to detect structural abnormalities in the fetus, chromosome screening (e.g. for Down's syndrome) and tests for infections in the mother that might affect the baby.

— Osteoporosis and osteomalacia —

Osteoporosis is a reduction in the total amount of bone tissue to the extent that the bones become weakened and liable to damage from normal mechanical stresses. It is the main underlying cause of fractured hip in elderly women. Bone mass reaches a peak around the third decade. In men it declines slowly and steadily thereafter. In women the rate of bone loss is much greater in the ten years following the menopause. Women also start off with less bone than men, and white people have less than people of Afro-Caribbean origin. A large proportion of elderly white women have lost sufficient bone to render them liable to fractures. Osteoporosis commonly presents as backache and a gradual loss of height due to squashing of the vertebrae or as a fracture of the hip associated with a fall (see chapter ten, page 226).

Factors other than the menopause that may also contribute to the earlier occurrence of osteoporosis are a lack of physical activity, smoking and excessive alcohol consumption. A number of medical conditions can cause osteoporosis. Corticosteroid therapy (e.g. prednisolone) and prolonged immobilisation (e.g. after stroke) also increase the rate of bone loss. Once established, osteoporosis is difficult to treat. For a healthier lifestyle to have maximum benefit it should be adopted as early as possible. Exercises intended to help maintain bone mass need to stress the weight bearing bones. Some particularly vigorous forms of aerobic exercise might actually be counterproductive in women. Good advice is required in this area. An adequate dietary intake of calcium is also important.

The most effective measure currently available for delaying the onset of osteoporosis is **hormone replacement therapy** (**HRT**) started at or soon after the menopause and continued for some years. Patients and drug regimens need to be carefully selected according to the clinical history. Some patients experience unpleasant side effects, but the consensus opinion is that many women benefit considerably from HRT. Accurate identification of those most at risk of osteoporosis would allow treatment to be offered to those most likely to benefit. There are some specialised tests capable of detecting osteoporosis at an early stage but they are not universally available.

A low level of calcium in the bones also causes bone weakness, pain and deformity. This is different to osteoporosis. It is called **rickets** in children and **osteomalacia** when it occurs in adults. It is usually due to a deficiency of **vitamin D**, a nutrient essential for normal calcium metabolism. Occasionally it is due to medical conditions which interfere with vitamin D or calcium metabolism. Most of our vitamin D is made in skin exposed to sunlight (ultraviolet light); some also comes from the diet. Vitamin D deficiency occurs when there is little or no exposure to sunlight and a lack of the vitamin in the diet. In the UK some Asian people and some elderly people living alone have been prone. Oral vitamin D supplements can be given to people at risk as a preventive measure. The recommended doses should not be exceeded because too much vitamin D can also be harmful.

9
TREATMENT

Basic considerations

Despite preventive medicine, people will still become ill and require treatment. Most of the work of hospitals is concerned with established disease. Medical or surgical treatment sometimes provides a complete cure. Often a disease or its effects can only be modified or controlled rather than completely eradicated (e.g. treatment of diabetes with insulin). The relief of distressing symptoms is also an important part of medical management; it may be the only treatment available. Medicines are often unnecessary when a disease is self-limiting and causes little damage or suffering. The excessive use of drugs in such circumstances can cause more problems than benefits. In the management of serious illness consideration is given not just to possible extension of life but also to the quality of life during and after treatment. The overall net benefits of treatments and their relative costs are major determinants in the allocation of limited health service funds.

Expert bodies frequently review the 'pros and cons' of different types of treatment and inform the medical profession through publications and letters. For instance, the British Medical Association and the Royal Pharmaceutical Society of Great Britain jointly publish twice yearly the *British National Formulary* which contains updated prescribing information and guidance for medical practitioners. Doctors exercise clinical judgment in individual cases. The variations in treatment regimens used in the management of some diseases, such as breast cancer, has led to national debate and even controversy. Measures taken to improve and co-ordinate approaches to complex disease management include the further education and training of doctors, the organisation of specialist treatment centres and the use of agreed protocols and clinical guidelines. The increasing use of audit to monitor results will also no doubt help to raise or maintain the standards of medical practice in general, providing it is medically rather than politically focused.

Good medical practice considers the whole person and not just their complaint or disease. Given the time constraints of a busy health service this can be difficult. Many practitioners manage to take the broader view and also inspire trust, confidence and a 'feel-better' factor in their patients, even before or without prescribing a medicine. Manner, approach and skills in communication and persuasion are all important. The role of supportive psychotherapy was mentioned in chapter five, page 134. These things not only help the patient to understand and come to terms with the disorder but they also encourage compliance with the treatment. These aspects are now receiving more attention in modern medical curricula.

Apart from doctors and nurses many other health professionals are involved in the overall medical care of the patient. Physiotherapy, occupational therapy and social services support may be particularly valuable during recovery and after the illness. Good communication between different health care teams is required to ensure continuity in the management of the patient, especially between hospital and general practice.

—— General supportive measures ——

The body has a remarkable ability to heal itself and repair the tissue damage caused by disease (and surgery). Good treatment assists this process. Apart from the therapy aimed specifically at the disease and the symptoms, care of the sick also involves a number of general supportive measures. Attention is given to comfort, hygiene, bodily functions and the prevention of problems in vulnerable areas such as the mouth and skin. Rest, physical activity, diet and fluid intake may require special consideration.

Rest

A good general rule is rest during the acute phase of a severe illness and a gradual increase in physical activity during the recovery phase, but the exact prescription depends upon the disease and the person. Complete rest is necessary during the acute or dangerous phases of some illnesses such as high fevers, rheumatic carditis, myocardial infarction and acute cardiac failure. However, too much bed rest can cause complications and a balance must be struck. Patients are now often gently mobilised within a few days of major surgery or an uncomplicated myocardial infarction in order to reduce the risk of thromboembolism. Prolonged immobilisation (e.g. after stroke) can lead to problems such as thrombosis in stagnant leg veins, weakening of bones and muscles, and pressure sores (chronic skin ulcers due to prolonged pressure at vulnerable sites on the body surface, commonly called bed sores). Good nursing can prevent or reduce some of these complications.

Diet and fluids

Some diseases require special diets. This may involve the restriction of certain dietary components, such as carbohydrate in diabetes (to help control plasma glucose levels) and protein in renal failure (to reduce the accumulation of nitrogen-containing substances, like urea). The diet must nevertheless contain adequate amounts of energy and essential nutrients. Prolonged illness sometimes leads to a nutritional deficiency state. Factors contributing to this include loss of appetite, poor diet, vomiting, loss of body substances (e.g. blood) and a catabolic state of metabolism (e.g. during infections and after major operations). The increased activities of the defence and repair systems increase the requirements for many nutrients (e.g. vitamin C). Nutrient deficiency can increase susceptibility to infection, impair wound healing and retard recovery from illness. A good diet during recovery and convalescence is particularly important.

Careful management of fluids is necessary when the patient's normal mechanisms for maintaining water and electrolyte homeostasis are compromised (e.g. in uncontrolled diabetes, coma, some renal diseases, and during and after major surgery). This is technically complex and requires considerable clinical competence. The balance of fluid intake (oral or intravenous) and output (e.g. urine, vomit, loss of blood, etc.) may need to be carefully monitored. Allowances are made for sweating (e.g. in fevers) and invisible water vapour losses from the skin and lungs. Regular weighing may be necessary. The replacement fluids are given by intravenous infusion when the oral route is inappropriate. The contents and the rate of the infusion must be carefully controlled to correct abnormal levels of water and electrolyte in the body, and to prevent overload of the circulatory system.

Unconscious or severely ill patients sometimes require feeding by special methods. This may involve passing liquid feeds into the stomach through a **nasogastric tube**, or intravenous feeding with specially prepared fluids containing essential nutrients.

—— Medicines - basic principles ——

Introduction

The therapeutically active ingredients in medicines, whether synthetically manufactured or extracted from natural materials such as plants, are chemicals. They all have molecular structures. Modern conventional medicines almost always contain precise amounts of pure ingredients whose nature, properties and actions have been well established by scientific methods. The discovery, development and manufacture of new medicines is difficult, time-consuming and very costly, and is virtually completely dependent on the existence of an innovative and effective pharmaceutical industry. Only a few of the thousands of promising new substances studied at the research phase pass all the necessary tests to allow them to enter clinical studies involving patients, and of those that do only a small proportion eventually find a useful place in clinical practice.

Before a medicine can be prescribed or sold it must normally have a product licence or authorisation from the appropriate government agency (e.g. Medicines Control Agency in the UK, Food and Drug Administration in the US). The licence number is on the product label or pack. A product licence may be granted if the company produces satisfactory evidence of product quality, safety and efficacy (effectiveness as a treatment). Quality refers to such things as the precise composition, levels of impurities, physical properties of the product, adequacy of manufacturing methods, determination of storage details and use-by dates, and the agreed limitations pertaining to all of these. The safety of a new medically active substance is usually tested in appropriate animal species (a requirement of licensing authorities) as well as in man. Animal toxicology data may not be required for new products containing well tried and tested substances, those that have been used in humans for many years without any obvious harm or serious side effects.

Efficacy must be studied in patients, usually in large carefully designed clinical trials, which also provide human safety data. All claims made for the medical benefits of a product and for its proposed therapeutic uses (**indications**) must be supported by evidence. Conventional medicines must normally satisfy the requirements for efficacy, safety and quality.

The situation has been different for many alternative medicine preparations which have in the past been subjected to less stringent scrutiny. However, there is now an increasing requirement that these products should at least be of good quality and safe in order to protect the consumer; new licensing arrangements are gradually coming into effect. Evidence of efficacy using conventionally accepted scientific methods may not be available for many alternative medicines. Without acceptable evidence of efficacy the medical claims that can be made for a product are limited.

In the UK there are three different legal categories of medical product licence:

1 **Prescription only medicines** (**POM**) must only be prescribed by registered doctors and dentists (and a few other qualified groups in special circumstances). They are usually dispensed by a registered pharmacist who will contact the

doctor if there appears to be a problem with the prescription;

2 **General Sales List** (**GSL**) medicines can be bought by the general public in retail pharmacies and in other stores such as supermarkets over the counter (**OTC**). Typical examples are simple cough, cold and headache remedies designed to relieve symptoms. Many contain aspirin or paracetamol, or both;

3 **Pharmacy sale** (**P**) medicines can only be purchased in a retail pharmacy under the supervision of a qualified pharmacist (e.g. hydrocortisone cream and ointment for certain skin conditions). There is currently a trend in the UK to deregulate more medicines from POM to P status, thus giving the consumer more freedom of choice, and the pharmacist more clinical responsibility.

Chemists give drugs chemical names which describe the molecular structure; they can be rather long. **Non-proprietary** or **generic** names are approved shortened versions. These names are not the property of any particular manufacturer. Thus, the generic name for the chemical N-acetyl-para-aminophenol is paracetamol (in the UK). The **brand** or **proprietary** name relates to a particular company. There are many brand names for products containing paracetamol; two well known ones are Panadol and Calpol. In general, the non-proprietary names are given in this book. Marketed products come in different forms (tablets, syrups, etc.) and contain a number of inactive ingredients, collectively known as **excipients**, to improve the general physical properties, acceptability (e.g. taste) and appearance of the medicine. Some products contain more than one active drug, especially many OTC products.

Pharmaceutical companies patent new potential drug molecules soon after discovery. By the time the product receives a licence for use as a medicine there may be little more than ten years of patent cover left. When the patent eventually expires other companies can manufacture and sell the drug. They too must apply for a product licence. Providing the indications and claims for the product and the recommended doses remain the same as those in the originator's licence, there is usually no need to supply additional efficacy and safety data in the application. But they must provide evidence of product quality. Additional data may be required when there are concerns about the consistency of movement of drug from the product into the body, such as a different rate of drug release or variable absorption of drug in the gut. This may necessitate a comparison with the originator's product in human volunteers to provide reassurance that the two products behave similarly, for instance give similar levels of drug in plasma (**bioequivalence study**).

The placebo effect

Belief in a treatment and the expectation that it will work can produce beneficial therapeutic effects. Patients sometimes experience pain relief if they believe their medicine contains a pain-relieving drug, even if it really contains no such drug. This is the **placebo effect** and the inactive medicine apparently producing it is known as a **placebo**. When possible, clinical trials on new drugs incorporate a comparison with a placebo, one group of patients receives the active and another the inactive preparation. These are often **double-blind** studies in which neither the person receiving nor the person administering the treatment know whether the medicine contains the active or inactive substance. This helps to eliminate subjective bias. A third party holds the code to drug allocation. The medicines must obviously appear similar; the inactive one is sometimes called a **dummy**. Such comparisons require careful study design and the application of specialised statistical methods. The active drug may be regarded as efficacious if it provides more benefit than placebo alone.

The placebo effect is psychological and it works best in conditions that are under strong mental influence (e.g. anxiety, pain). However, it can produce physical effects in the body. Some people are much more susceptible to the placebo effect than others. Those that are tend to have certain characteristics, such as being generally more open to suggestion.

How drugs work

The drug substance producing the medically useful effect inside the body is often chemically identical to the drug originally administered to the patient (parent drug), but not always. Metabolism in the liver changes the chemical structure of many drugs – the resultant chemical products are known as **metabolites**. Sometimes drug metabolites are responsible for the therapeutic response. The parent drug or the metabolites can cause unwanted effects too. In the rest of this section the term drug refers to the **therapeutically active** substance.

Drugs act by modifying chemical processes. The initial event is often a selective interaction ('lock and key' principle again) with a protein that has a specific and important role (e.g. enzyme, receptor). The drug alters the normal activity of the protein and this ultimately leads to a biological response. The chain of events is generally complex. The final effect may be to damage an organism or cell (e.g. antimicrobial and anticancer drugs) or to modify an undesirable physiological state favourably (e.g. reduce high blood pressure).

The **penicillins** and **cephalosporins** are groups of drugs that kill particular bacteria by interfering with the manufacture of the bacterial cell wall. Other antimicrobial drugs act by interfering with microbial DNA synthesis (e.g. the antibacterial **trimethoprim**, the antiviral **acyclovir**) or protein synthesis (e.g. **erythromycin** and the **tetracyclines**).

Most drugs used to produce physiological adjustments act on cell receptors. These receptors normally initiate cellular changes in response to interactions with natural chemical messengers (e.g. histamine, adrenaline). They are critical in the regulation of cellular activities. There are many different types of receptor, each responding to a specific messenger, and some occur only in particular types of cell. Drugs that act on receptors mimic some of the properties of the natural messenger. They compete for molecular interaction with the receptor. Some drugs activate the receptors and induce a response similar to that normally produced by the messenger (**agonists**). Others block the messenger molecule, the natural agonist, but are unable themselves to activate the receptor (**antagonists**), thus causing a net reduction in the physiological response. The following important examples illustrate some of these principles.

Beta receptors

The natural hormone **adrenaline**, from the adrenal gland (see chapter five, page 125), can act on receptors in the lung and cause the muscles in the bronchial wall to relax. This dilates the airways and makes breathing easier. Adrenaline also stimulates receptors in the heart muscle causing an increase in the rate and strength of the heart beat. These responses normally come into play in fight and flight situations. The particular receptors involved are known as **beta receptors**. Those in the heart are **beta$_1$ receptors** and those in the lung are **beta$_2$ receptors**. Beta-agonist drugs have been developed which selectively activate beta$_2$ receptors. Some are particularly useful in the treatment of asthma because they can make breathing easier without too much stimulation of the heart (a potentially dangerous effect). An example of a selective **beta$_2$-agonist** is **salbutamol** which can be given via an inhaler (well known brand name is Ventolin). Beta-antagonists (**beta-blockers**) on the other hand are useful in the treatment of hypertension due to their blockade of beta$_1$ receptors. The mechanism by which they reduce high blood pressure is not fully understood but initially it is by reducing cardiac output. Some beta-blockers have a more selective action against beta$_1$ than beta$_2$ receptors and some also partially stimulate receptors. Thus different types of beta-blocker produce slightly different effects. None are completely selective. Beta-blockers are potentially dangerous in people with asthma. Neither should they be given to people who may be at risk from a reduction in cardiac output (e.g. those prone to heart failure).

Histamine receptors

There are two types of histamine receptor, H$_1$, and H$_2$. H$_1$-antagonist drugs are the antihistamines commonly used in the treatment of hay fever and other allergic reactions. The formation of acid in the stomach is increased when locally produced histamine stimulates the H$_2$-receptors on the parietal cells (see chapter 3, page 104). Excessive acid secretion can be controlled with H$_2$-antagonist drugs such as **cimetidine** and **ranitidine**, which are useful in the treatment of peptic ulcer.

Drugs can also be made more selective by other means. For instance, some of the newer antihistamines tend to cause less drowsiness because their molecules are drawn to watery environments rather than the lipid rich regions of the brain.

How the body handles drugs

Most drugs designed to be taken by mouth are efficiently absorbed into the body from the gastro-intestinal tract. Like many nutrients they must first travel in the portal vein to the liver before passing into the general blood circulation. The vascular system then rapidly distributes the drug around the body and to its site of action in an organ or tissue.

Metabolism in the liver (and occasionally in other tissues) converts many drugs into metabolites. Rapid metabolic conversion in the liver may drastically reduce the amount of parent drug reaching the general circulation – the so-called **first pass effect**. The metabolism of some drugs is slower but may continue during general recirculation through the liver. One of the liver's main functions is to remove molecules that are toxic or foreign to the body. Drug metabolism often inactivates the drug and makes it more water soluble, so that the kidney can remove it from the body. Some drugs are designed to resist metabolism.

Poor absorption from the gastro-intestinal tract reduces the amount of drug entering the general circulation and therefore the amount available for therapeutic activity (i.e. **bioavailability** is reduced). The presence of food in the gastro-intestinal tract can affect the bioavailability of some drugs, for better or worse.

The kidney removes drug substances from the body by excreting them into the urine. Drugs that assume a fat soluble form in the body (i.e. molecules that are drawn to fats and organic solvents rather than water) cross cell membranes more readily and may be reabsorbed back into the body from the renal tubules. The metabolites are often more water soluble and are more likely to pass into the urine.

After dosing, the drug passes into the general circulation and the plasma drug concentration rises. But the drug is continually being removed by the liver and/or kidneys. The drug concentration therefore rises to a peak value and then gradually declines, until the next dose is given. The rate of decline of the drug concentration in plasma is sometimes expressed in terms of a **half-life**. This is the time taken for a drug to halve its concentration in plasma. For instance, if a drug has a half-life of two hours the level will halve every two hours, so that after, say, six hours the level will be only one-eighth of the original concentration. The half-life is only an approximation of the behaviour of many drugs but it can be useful in the determination of the dosage schedule (e.g. time between doses). Too frequent dosing can lead to excessive accumulation of a drug in the body.

The recommended dose and frequency of dosing, and the duration of drug treatment are determined by efficacy and safety studies and by studies of drug levels in the body. Drugs are taken by mouth in the form of tablets, capsules, solutions and suspensions (different **formulations**). New formulations sometimes require additional studies because of possible bioavailability problems. Some formulations are designed to release a drug slowly in order to provide sustained plasma concentrations and less frequent dosing.

There are of course other ways to administer drugs. Those that are poorly bioavailable can sometimes be given by injection. A few drugs are adequately absorbed from a patch applied to the skin (e.g. nicotine) or from a small tablet placed under the tongue (e.g. **glyceryl trinitrate** for the relief of angina pectoris). These manoeuvres also avoid the first pass effect because the drug goes straight into the general circulation.

Drugs are also injected or given by intravenous infusion when a quick response is required, or when it is imperative that adequate or very precise drug levels are maintained in the body, or when drugs cannot be given by mouth. Great care must be taken to ensure that drugs are not given too rapidly by the intravenous route because of the possibility of transient very high concentrations causing dangerous acute toxicity in vital organs such as the heart and brain.

Special dose adjustments are made for children according to age or body size. Sometimes allowances are also made for differences in the sizes of adults. Many factors can affect drug action and there are often large variations in the way individuals handle and respond to drugs. For instance, the rate of removal of a drug from the body may be reduced in the elderly and in patients with liver or kidney disease. In such cases the standard adult dosage regimen may lead to accumulation of a drug in the body and unwanted side effects.

Unwanted drug effects

Drugs sometimes produce unwanted and unfavourable effects, generally known as **adverse reactions** or side effects. Details of the common and important adverse reactions are available in pharmaceutical company **data sheets** and official publications supplied to prescribing doctors, and in **patient information leaflets**. At first sight the lists of warnings and possible side effects can be daunting, even terrifying. It is important to keep a sense of perspective. The potent drugs with a greater propensity for adverse reactions are more likely to be used in the treatment of serious illness. The probable benefits of treatment must be balanced against the possible risks and disadvantages – the essence of clinical judgment. For most of the drugs in common use serious adverse reactions are rare and the commoner side effects mild. Symptoms commonly attributed to drugs are nausea, headaches and tiredness. Many drugs can indeed cause such symptoms, but so can many of the diseases they are used to treat, and some healthy volunteers receiving placebo in double-blind trials may also experience similar effects. Therefore, one cannot always attribute the adverse event to the active drug.

Some adverse reactions are an extension of the therapeutic action of the drug and can therefore be anticipated. For instance, a drug that kills cancer cells may also attack normal, actively proliferating bone marrow cells and cause **neutropenia** (low white blood cell count), which, if unchecked, is potentially dangerous. The white blood cell count is therefore monitored regularly during cancer chemotherapy. Drugs with potent therapeutic effects on receptors in the heart are also capable of producing unwanted and sometimes dangerous cardiac events when the therapeutic dose is exceeded. These types of adverse reaction can be minimised by regular patient monitoring and careful dose adjustment. When the dose causing adverse effects is not much greater than that required for therapeutic benefit, the drug is said to have a low **therapeutic index**.

Many of the commonly used antibacterials, antihistamines and pain-relieving drugs have relatively high therapeutic indices. Nevertheless, even with these drugs it can be dangerous to exceed the recommended dose. For instance, a large dose of paracetamol can produce severe liver damage and requires urgent treatment.

Some individuals have a particular sensitivity to a drug (**idiosyncrasy**). This may be an allergic or toxic reaction and there may be a genetic predisposition. Unfortunately, in most instances susceptible individuals cannot yet be identified in advance of treatment, unless of course they have already experienced such reactions from previous drug therapy. Many drugs produce skin rashes in susceptible people (e.g. penicillins). Very occasionally these are severe and associated with a more generalised drug-induced illness. This is one of the reasons why sulphonamides are now used much less frequently. Administration of a penicillin-like drug to someone who has already been strongly sensitized to penicillin from a previous treatment can result in anaphylaxis (see chapter three, page 94). Awareness of a history of drug hypersensitivity is most important.

A drug may have been studied in a few thousand patients before the grant of a product licence. This provides useful information about the commoner adverse reactions. However, tens or even hundreds of thousands of patients must be studied to pick up rare, but sometimes severe, idiosyncratic reactions. There are special schemes for continually monitoring adverse effects after the grant of the licence. Occasionally drugs are withdrawn from the market, either by the manufacturer or the regulatory authority, because of unacceptable adverse reactions.

Sometimes drugs cause problems by interacting adversely with other drugs. This is a vast and complicated subject requiring considerable vigilance on the part of the manufacturer, regulatory authority, prescribing doctor, dispensing pharmacist, and the patient. Patients need to be aware of the contents of the OTC medicines they purchase and should discuss with the pharmacist or doctor the possibility of interactions with other medicines they may be taking.

Elderly patients are at particular risk of adverse reactions because they often have more than one ailment, are often taking more than one drug simultaneously and their bodies handle drugs less efficiently than younger people.

The treatment of selected cardiovascular disorders

The following sections introduce more drugs and therapeutic principles. They are not complete accounts of the treatment of these disorders.

Essential hypertension

Severe hypertension requires urgent treatment. The management of less severe hypertension depends on the diastolic and systolic blood pressures, the presence or absence of complications (e.g. changes in the retina) and whether or not treatable predisposing factors are present. A high alcohol intake, a high salt intake and obesity may contribute to high blood pressure. Weight control and a reduction in alcohol and salt intake sometimes help to control mild hypertension without the need to resort to drug treatment.

When drugs are required, diuretics or beta-blockers are usually the first choice. **Diuretics** remove water from the body by reducing water reabsorption in the kidney. They increase urine output (diuresis). How they maintain the anti-hypertensive effect is not known. A small dose of a relatively weak diuretic (e.g. **bendrofluazide**) is often sufficient to control hypertension. Sometimes a combination of a diuretic and a beta-blocker may be necessary. A number of other drug treatment options are available for more resistant hypertension.

Heart failure

Diuretics are also useful in the treatment of heart failure. They reduce the fluid load on the heart, remove excess water from the lungs and reduce oedema. Sometimes powerful diuretics are needed (e.g. **frusemide**).

Drugs known as **ACE-inhibitors** are beneficial in the long-term treatment of chronic heart failure. Treatment with ACE-inhibitors is often initiated in hospital under careful medical supervision. ACE stands for **angiotensin converting enzyme**, an enzyme responsible for the formation of an important chemical messenger called **angiotensin II**. Angiotensin II acts on the smooth muscle in blood vessels, causing them to constrict, and it also stimulates the cortex of the adrenal gland to release the hormone **aldosterone**, which in turn stimulates the renal tubule to retain sodium (and therefore water) in the body. This is all part of a normal homeostatic control system. In heart failure the control setting is altered – some blood vessels are narrowed and water and salt is retained, events which increase the workload on the heart. ACE-inhibitors such as **captopril** and **enalapril** block the formation of angiotensin II and thereby reverse these effects. ACE-inhibitors are also known as **vasodilators**. They are sometimes used to treat hypertension.

Other drugs may be required to control heart failure. Digoxin, a chemical extracted from foxglove leaves, was once commonly used but is now less favoured, except in particular circumstances.

Myocardial infarction (MI)

Patients with suspected MI are usually transferred rapidly to a hospital coronary care unit because of the possibility of sudden dangerous complications and the need for continuous ECG monitoring. **Morphine** is often given by injection immediately after the attack to relieve pain and anxiety, and is usually very effective. Because morphine can cause nausea and vomiting an **anti-emetic** (a drug that prevents vomiting) is often given at the same time. When complications such as heart failure, shock and arrhythmias occur after MI they require very specialised treatment. **Fibrinolytic drugs** (e.g. **streptokinase**, **alteplase**) activate the plasma system that degrades (lyses) fibrin. In suitable patients, intravenous administration of these agents can lyse thrombi in the coronary arteries and thereby lessen the damage to the heart. This therapy must be started soon after MI, preferably within three hours.

Small daily oral doses of aspirin started soon after MI can reduce the likelihood of a second attack by reducing the ability of platelets to clump. For similar reasons aspirin is also used in the management of many patients with angina or a history of transient ischaemic attacks or stroke. Such treatment should always be under medical supervision because of the possibility of unwanted effects.

——— The treatment of cancer ———

This section concentrates on the methods used to eradicate cancer cells from the body. There are three types of treatment: **surgery**, **radiotherapy** and **chemotherapy** (drugs). They may be used singly or in various combinations depending on the cancer and its stage, and the state of the patient.

Surgery

Surgical eradication of localised cancer involves removal of the visible tumour together with a surrounding area of apparently normal tissue. Sometimes the surgery is extended to include removal of the lymph nodes draining the area. Surgery is the definitive curative treatment for many tumours at an early stage. The use of radiotherapy and/or chemotherapy in addition to surgery can further improve the prognosis of some cancers.

In the past, many surgeons favoured very extensive surgery for early (localised) breast cancer, believing that this would provide the best chance of a complete cure. This approach involves complete removal of the breast, other adjacent tissues and the associated lymph nodes. Recent clinical trials suggest that much simpler and less disfiguring operations (e.g. removing the lump but conserving the breast) combined with radiotherapy of the local lymph nodes produce similar survival rates. Accurate staging of the tumour is important and this usually necessitates the removal of some lymph nodes. There are still differences in approach, and views will continue to change as new evidence becomes available. Patients need to be aware of the options available to them.

Surgery usually aims to cure cancer but sometimes it is palliative, providing symptomatic relief rather than a cure. For instance, surgical intervention is indicated when a carcinoma obstructs the passage of material in the bowel, even if the cancer is at an advanced stage and there is little chance of a cure.

Radiotherapy

Radiotherapy is the treatment of disease with **ionising radiation**. This type of radiation kills cancer cells by damaging their DNA. It is less effective in the presence of the low oxygen concentrations that may occur in the deeper regions of large tumours. Radiotherapy is often used to relieve bone pain caused by metastases. Normal cells are also vulnerable to the effects of radiation. A number of measures are taken to ensure that radiotherapy damages the tumour cells more than the normal cells and that vital tissues are protected. For instance, the beam of radiation can be aimed from different positions outside the body so that an internal tumour deposit receives more radiation than the tissues surrounding it. Accurate location of the tumour and careful positioning of the patient are essential in such cases. Radiotherapy often involves attendance several days each week for a few weeks.

Chemotherapy

Cancer chemotherapy is the administration of drugs to eradicate cancer cells. **Cytotoxic drugs** kill cells by interfering with vital biochemical processes such as DNA synthesis or replication. They attack actively proliferating tumour cells; those in the resting phase are relatively resistant. Treatment schedules are designed to reduce the number of malignant cells significantly after each dose and to catch the dormant cells when they emerge from the resting phase. The smaller the initial total number of malignant cells and the larger the proportion of actively dividing cells, the greater the likelihood of complete eradication. Unfortunately, residual cancer cells sometimes persist after treatment and mutations can develop resistance to anticancer drugs. Cytotoxic drugs also attack normal tissues containing actively dividing cells, especially the bone marrow (site of new blood cell production), gastro-intestinal tract epithelium and the skin. Therefore common unwanted effects of cancer chemotherapy are neutropenia and other blood disorders, gastro-intestinal upsets such as nausea and vomiting, and hair loss (usually temporary). The adverse reactions vary according to the type of anticancer drug used. Achievement of an adequate therapeutic effect almost inevitably involves some damage to normal tissues. The aim is to maximally damage the cancer without causing irreversible damage to normal vital tissues. Blood cell counts are monitored regularly and therapy is adjusted appropriately. Destruction of all or most of the cancer cells often requires a long course of treatment. Treatment with a combination of cytotoxic drugs with different actions sometimes improves the selective killing of malignant cells. Tumours vary considerably in their response.

Chemotherapy produces remarkably good cure rates in some of the less common forms of cancer (e.g. **acute lymphoblastic leukaemia** in childhood, and **Hodgkin's disease**). It also improves the prognosis of some cancers when used as a back up to surgery (e.g. breast and ovarian cancer). Chemotherapy often induces **remissions**, apparent disease-free periods, in patients with advanced cancer. This can often usefully extend life even though a complete cure is unlikely. Cancer treatment is the subject of a large number of clinical trials under the auspices of various national and international bodies. Progress is inevitably slow but major advances have been made.

Sex hormones stimulate the growth of some tumours (e.g. breast, prostate). Removal of the influence of these hormones can inhibit tumour growth and considerably delay progression of the disease. The malignant cells in many patients with breast cancer have oestrogen receptors on their surface. **Tamoxifen** is an oestrogen-receptor antagonist drug which can increase survival in many patients with oestrogen-dependent breast cancer.

Short monographs on selected drugs

Antibacterial drugs

Some of the biochemical features of bacteria differ markedly from those of human cells. This facilitates the development of antibacterials with a high therapeutic index.

Factors that influence the choice of drug for the treatment of a bacterial infection include its known antibacterial activity (the bugs normally susceptible to its action), its ability to penetrate to the site of infection (e.g. intracellular bacteria; infections of brain, bone, etc.), the proposed route of administration (injections or intravenous infusions may be preferable in severe infections) and its side effects. Many bacteria are now resistant to a variety of antibacterials. Prescribing policy tends to change from time to time because of the emergence of new drug resistance patterns, the wish to hold some drugs in reserve for special situations, reports of adverse reactions and economic considerations. The choice of antibacterial therapy also depends on the characteristics of the individual patient (e.g. allergy, immune status, child, pregnancy, renal failure). Some infections, such as tuberculosis, require combination chemotherapy with two or more drugs at the same time; this can reduce the emergence of resistant strains. Compliance with recommended treatment schedules is important. They are designed to give the best chances of a cure.

Antibacterials are less likely to be effective if a large focus of infection persists. Abscesses require surgical drainage and dirty wounds must be cleaned. Patients with urinary tract infections are often advised to drink plenty of water to ensure a good urine flow, and to empty the bladder regularly and completely.

There are many types of antibacterial drug, and generally more than one type is available for any particular infection. We shall consider just one class of antibacterials in more detail, the penicillins. **Penicillin G** (or **benzylpenicillin**) was the first available. It is active against streptococci, treponema pallidum (the organism responsible for syphilis), meningococcus (one cause of meningitis) and a few other bacteria. It is broken down in the stomach and must therefore be given by injection. Long acting injectable forms are used for the treatment of syphilis. **Penicillin V** has a similar spectrum of activity but it can be taken by mouth. It is often used to treat streptococcal tonsillitis. However, its absorption from the gut is variable and it is not used for infections where inadequate plasma concentrations could have serious consequences.

Staphylococcus aureus is responsible for a number of serious infections, especially in hospitals, and the organism is now almost always resistant to the action of penicillin G and V. This is because it produces penicillinase, an enzyme which breaks a critical part of the penicillin molecule. Penicillins such as **cloxacillin** and **flucloxacillin** are usually resistant and are used specifically to treat infections due to penicillinase-producing Staphylococci. Strains resistant to these drugs have appeared in a few hospitals.

Ampicillin is effective against a wider range of bacteria than the above penicillins and is therefore known as a **broad-spectrum antibiot**ic. It is commonly used for the treatment of chronic bronchitis and urinary tract infections. Penicillinases inactivate ampicillin and more bacteria are becoming resistant to the drug. Ampicillin can be taken by mouth but its absorption is not ideal. **Amoxycillin** is similar to ampicillin but it is better absorbed. Sometimes amoxycillin is given together with a substance that inhibits penicillinases. There are other penicillins with different properties. The penicillins have been and still are of great value in the treatment of certain infections. Other types of antibacterial agents are available for use in people with penicillin allergy which, unfortunately, is not uncommon.

Antiviral drugs

The development of highly selective antiviral drugs has been more difficult because viruses utilise biochemical mechanisms inside the human cell. There have been some notable successes.

Acyclovir is effective in the treatment of herpes virus infections, such as genital herpes and shingles, and is relatively non-toxic. It can be life-saving in patients with herpes encephalitis and in immune-compromised patients (i.e. normal body defences not working) with herpes virus infections.

Zidovudine (**AZT**) is active against HIV. It can prolong the life of patients with AIDS but does not cure the condition. Therapeutic doses can cause anaemia and neutropenia which require careful monitoring. The virus can develop resistance to zidovudine.

Acyclovir and zidovudine selectively interfere with the formation of viral DNA. They inhibit rather than destroy the viruses.

Analgesics and anti-inflammatory drugs

Analgesics are drugs that reduce sensitivity to pain. They can be divided into opioid and non-opioid types. **Opioid analgesics** produce their effects by activating specific receptors in the central nervous system. These receptors naturally interact with **opioid peptides** (peptides are very short pieces of protein chain – they contain just a few amino acids), substances formed in the body and which have an important role in pain regulation. Strong opioid analgesics such as **morphine** and **diamorphine** (**heroin**) are used to relieve moderate to severe pain, particularly of the type associated with some diseases of internal organs. Prolonged use can lead to dependence and tolerance (see chapter five, page 132) but this does not obviate their use in appropriate medical circumstances. Oral formulations of morphine are extremely valuable in the control of pain in terminally ill patients. **Pethidine** is a rapidly but short acting opioid analgesic commonly used to relieve labour pain. Weak opioid analgesics, such as **codeine**, are used for mild to moderate pain. There are many opioid analgesics, and they all have side effects; the choice depends on the clinical situation.

Most non-opioid analgesics are also anti-inflammatory drugs. An exception is **paracetamol**, which is a very useful drug for the relief of mild to moderate pain not associated with inflammation. Great care must be taken not to exceed the recommended dose of paracetamol – high doses can cause dangerous liver damage. **Aspirin** and a number of other drugs (e.g. **ibuprofen**, **naproxen**) have both anti-inflammatory and analgesic actions. A distinction is made between these and the anti-inflammatory steroids and they are given the general title of **non-steroidal anti-inflammatory drugs** (**NSAIDs**). NSAIDs are useful in the treatment of many painful joint and muscle disorders, including osteoarthritis and rheumatoid arthritis. Aspirin is a useful analgesic but the doses required to produce good anti-inflammatory effects are high and likely to cause side effects. Aspirin often causes gastrointestinal upsets. In the UK it is recommended that children under 12 years should not be given aspirin because of its possible role in the development of **Reye's syndrome**, a rare but serious disorder of the liver and brain. In general, NSAIDs are avoided when there is a history of peptic ulceration or of certain allergic reactions. They sometimes make asthma worse. They must also be used with caution in the elderly.

Certain steroid drugs have powerful anti-inflammatory properties and are very important in the treatment of several diseases. These drugs are variously called corticosteroids, glucocorticoids and often, misleadingly, just steroids. In fact, the basic steroid chemical structure, the core of which consists of rings of carbon atoms, is common to many substances with quite different properties and functions, such as cholesterol, bile acids, sex hormones (e.g. oestrogens in women, testosterone in men) and aldosterone and hydrocortisone from the adrenal cortex. Hydrocortisone has anti-inflammatory properties and also affects glucose metabolism. A number of synthetic derivatives (e.g. **prednisolone**) have even more potent anti-inflammatory effects. The term 'steroid therapy' often refers to treatment with anti-inflammatory drugs such as prednisolone. Hormone replacement therapy (HRT) is quite different and refers to treatment with drugs having the properties of certain female sex hormones (they also have the basic steroid structure).

Anti-inflammatory steroids suppress inflammation and the immune response. They are often used in the treatment of severe asthma and rheumatoid arthritis, and also to suppress the immune system after transplantation in order to help prevent rejection of the donor organ. Although they can be extremely effective, and sometimes life-saving, these drugs also produce many side effects, especially at the higher doses and when taken for long periods. They also interfere with the normal hypothalamic-pituitary-adrenal cortex control system (see chapter five, page 125) and affect normal hydrocortisone production. This effect may last for many months after the cessation of treatment and patients may respond poorly to severe stress situations (trauma, surgery, infection). Steroid therapy is usually withdrawn gradually rather than stopped abruptly. Patients who are on or have recently been on anti-inflammatory steroids usually carry information cards for use in emergencies. They may require additional corticosteroid cover in stress situations.

Anaesthetics

Anaesthetics are substances that produce a loss of sensation, especially pain. Local anaesthetics temporarily block the conduction of signals in sensory nerve fibres, thereby producing loss of sensation in a particular part of the body. General anaesthetics affect the brain and can produce a loss of awareness as well as a general loss of pain sensation. Deep anaesthesia relaxes muscles, which can be useful to the surgeon. However, it may also suppress vital activities such as breathing, which may require special assistance. Modern surgical anaesthesia tends to be light, but enough to produce loss of awareness; separate drugs are used to relax the muscles. The drugs used to maintain general anaesthesia are usually administered as a gas through a mask or breathing tube. A common anaesthetic gas mixture contains **nitrous oxide** and **halothane**. Obviously, it is important that sufficient oxygen is supplied too. At the very lightest level the sensation of pain may be diminished without loss of consciousness. Nitrous oxide on its own is a relatively weak anaesthetic. A 50 per cent mixture of nitrous oxide in oxygen (**Entonox**) is often used as an analgesic in childbirth and at the scene of accidents.

10
SURGERY

This chapter provides only a very brief and superficial excursion into the world of surgery.

Who does what?

Surgery is divided into a number of separate disciplines, each with its own consultants. **Orthopaedics** is the branch specialising in bone and joint disorders. **Gynaecology** deals with disorders of the female reproductive system; it is usually combined with **obstetrics**, which is concerned with the medical and surgical aspects of pregnancy and childbirth. Other surgical specialities are **eye** surgery, **ear, nose and throat** (**ENT**) surgery, **plastic** surgery, **paediatric** surgery (children), **urology** (kidneys and urinary tract), **cardiothoracic** surgery (chest) and **neurosurgery**. **General surgery** is the separate and more common branch of surgery that deals with a wide variety of disorders not usually covered by the other specialisms. General surgeons operate on many of the abdominal organs and other parts of the body. Typically their repertoire includes such things as breast, stomach, bowel and pancreatic tumours, peptic ulcers, gall bladder disorders, some thyroid disorders, hernias, circumcisions, varicose veins, piles and acute abdominal emergencies such as appendicitis and bowel obstruction.

— Surgical vocabulary and procedures —

The removal of a part (**excision**) is denoted by the suffix **-ecto-my**. Thus, **mastectomy**, **gastrectomy**, **colectomy**, **appendicectomy** and **haemorrhoidectomy** refer to excision of the breast, stomach, colon, appendix and piles respectively. **Resection** is the surgical removal of part of an organ or tissue (e.g. removal of a portion of bowel containing a tumour). The cutting of a part (**incision**) with a surgical knife (scalpel) is designated by the suffix **-tomy**. **Laparotomy** and **thoracotomy** refer to incisions through the abdominal and chest walls respectively. **Vagotomy** is the cutting of the vagus nerves. The suffix **-stomy** refers to the surgical creation of an artificial opening. A **colostomy** is the formation of an opening from the large bowel onto the body surface; it functions as an artificial anus. It may be required to relieve intestinal obstruction (sometimes as a temporary measure) or when the rectum and anus require removal because of a carcinoma.

The damage arising from incision, excision and resection requires very careful repair to ensure proper healing and minimal scar formation. **Sutures** are threads (e.g. catgut, silk, wire) used to stitch the cut edges together. **Ligatures** are threads drawn around ducts or blood vessels to prevent unwanted leakage. Sometimes a tube (drain) is left temporarily in the operation wound to provide drainage to the outside to prevent internal pooling of fluid. Surgery often involves biological plumbing, such as the removal and relief of an obstruction in a duct, tract or vessel, or the formation of an **anastomosis**, a connection between two tubes (e.g. between the cut ends remaining after bowel resection).

The surgical operation – before, during and after

There is much more to surgery than the operation itself. The skill and experience of the surgeon is generally more than adequate to ensure a good chance of technical success. When problems do arise from surgery they are often of a medical nature and tend to occur in the period after the operation (**postoperative**). Major surgery is a severe assault on the body and it causes a shock-like state and increased catabolism (breakdown of the body's own tissues). Everything possible must be done before, during and after the operation to minimise shock, prevent complications and aid recovery. This includes relieving pain and making the patient comfortable.

Surgery requires a great deal of organisation and interdisciplinary co-operation. In the hospital the surgical houseman (house surgeon) is usually responsible for organising and co-ordinating the medical care of the patient. A well-run unit will provide as smooth a passage as possible for the patient from before admission to hospital until recovery is complete. This requires continuous attention to surgical and medical management and to the needs of the patient as a person. Good communication with all involved, patient, relatives and professionals, is essential. The patient should receive a clear explanation of the proposed treatment, its purpose and risks, what to expect at the various stages and the likely outcome. They will be asked to sign an operation consent form which permits the surgeon to carry out the specified operation. Some operations result in particular psychological and physical difficulties for the patient (e.g. mastectomy, colostomy, amputation). Such cases require exceptionally good counselling and expert professional and technical support, which should be available.

Emergency surgery must often be undertaken in less than ideal circumstances. The patient may already be very ill and debilitated and infection may be present. Intensive medical treatment may be required to reduce the increased risk from surgical treatment in such circumstances. Patients are generally fitter and better prepared for elective non-urgent (cold) surgery which can be undertaken at a more appropriate time. Even so, many are not fit, some suffer from medical conditions, and the elderly are generally at greater risk from anaesthesia and surgery. The patient may be reassessed and the prudence of surgery reconfirmed a short while before the proposed date of admission to hospital. The house surgeon and the anaesthetist examine the patient after admission, often on the day before the operation. Sometimes particular preparations and precautions are necessary, such as: antibiotic cover, adjustment of current medication, availability of blood for transfusion during surgery, insertion of an intravenous line, cleansing of the gut before bowel surgery, etc. Before the operation the patient's identity is double-checked and the surgeon often marks the skin at the proposed site of operation with an indelible pen to help avoid mistakes.

During anaesthesia there is a risk of inhaling stomach contents. Therefore patients are not allowed food or drink for some hours before the operation. Drugs (e.g. **diazepam**, **lorazepam**) are usually administered shortly before the operation to allay anxiety (**premedication**). Anaesthesia is initiated in an anteroom adjoining the operating theatre. In the UK, **anaesthetics** is a distinct medical discipline with its own consultants. A drug (e.g. thiopentone) is given intravenously to produce rapid unconsciousness (**induction**). Anaesthesia is then maintained by means of anaesthetic gases (see chapter nine, page 218). The anaesthetist controls the various devices necessary for life support during the operation. To reduce adverse effects and allow more complex surgery, anaesthesia is usually maintained at a relatively light level, enough to abolish pain and awareness; muscle relaxing drugs may be given to reduce muscle tone and movement, and the patient's respiration may be supported by a mechanical ventilator; this is modern **balanced anaesthesia**. Artificial ventilation requires the insertion of a special tube into the trachea, usually via the mouth. A small balloon cuff surrounding the main tube is inflated to hug the wall of the trachea; this prevents gas leakage around the tube and it also prevents unwanted secretions and debris in the throat from entering the lungs. The tracheal tube is usually inserted soon after induction. Sometimes surgery can be performed under local anaesthetic, with the patient conscious but sedated.

The many rituals of the operating theatre are designed to protect the patient from infection, haemorrhage and unnecessary damage. Bacterial contamination is reduced by disinfection of surfaces and skin, by pumping clean air into the theatre and by aseptic technique, which aims to prevent spread of infection to the patient. The latter includes the use of sterile instruments, and sterile drapes, gowns, gloves, masks and caps to cover the germ-shedding areas of the body. Good surgical technique ensures that clean areas are not contaminated by dirty materials or instruments. Extra special precautions are warranted in orthopaedic surgery because bone infection can be particularly troublesome. Theatres may require thorough decontamination after an operation on an infected patient; such cases are often left until the end of the operating session.

For the first hour or two after the operation the patient is carefully monitored and nursed in the **recovery room** until stabilised and conscious. During this period normal breathing is established and specific therapeutic regimens may be instituted (e.g. treatment for postoperative pain, intravenous fluids). Depending on the circumstances, the patient may then be transferred back to the surgical ward, to an intensive care unit with specialised equipment and a high staff to patient ratio, or in some hospitals to an intermediary 'high dependency' unit.

Important complications that can occur in the days following a major operation include haemorrhage, lung collapse, wound infection, deep vein thrombosis and pulmonary embolism. Blockage of segments of the lungs by mucus is a common cause of pulmonary collapse after surgery under general anaesthesia; this is a treatable condition, more common in smokers. The elderly are more prone to pneumonia after major surgery. The process leading to deep vein thrombosis and pulmonary embolism often starts in the theatre. A number of measures can be taken pre-operatively, during the operation and postoperatively to reduce the likelihood of most of these complications. Most people now recover from major surgery without serious complications and without too much discomfort.

—— Selected surgical topics ——

Minimal access surgery

Traditionally, many surgical operations have required large incisions in the body wall to provide the surgeon with adequate visibility and room for manipulation. In some circumstances too small an opening can be imprudent (e.g. if heavy internal bleeding is a possibility). New technologies and modern surgical techniques now make it possible to conduct more operations through very small openings in the body wall or via body orifices. This important development is variously known as **minimal access surgery**, **minimally invasive surgery** or commonly as 'keyhole surgery'.

Some branches of surgery have used such techniques for many years. For instance, gynaecologists often perform female sterilisation by **laparoscopy**, a technique in which a special endoscope is inserted into the peritoneal cavity through a small hole in the abdominal wall. The abdominal cavity is inflated with a gas to facilitate visualisation of the internal organs with the instrument's optical system. The surgeon operates by remotely controlling small surgical instruments at the end of the laparoscope. Examples of operations that have traditionally involved substantial incisions but which are now often amenable to minimal access surgery are appendicectomy, hernia repairs and some gall bladder operations. Orthopaedic surgeons are using these techniques for operations inside joint spaces, and neurosurgeons sometimes use them in order to reduce unwanted damage to important areas of the brain. Some instruments have small electronic cameras which can relay images from inside the body to a screen in the operating theatre. The surgeon operates via the endoscope using small and increasingly sophisticated remotely controlled instruments.

Advantages of minimal access surgery are less tissue damage and less blood loss (which decreases the shock effect on the body), less postoperative pain, a shorter stay in hospital, quicker recovery and a better cosmetic result. Complications occurring during the operation may present more difficulties for the surgeon. Sometimes it is necessary to convert minimal access into more conventional open surgery.

Minimal access surgery requires special facilities and the surgeons need to develop new skills. There have been some concerns regarding the responsibilities and arrangements for training surgeons and for ensuring adequate and consistent standards of practice in this rapidly expanding area.

Day surgery

Improved surgical techniques, such as minimal access surgery, changes in medical opinions and strategies, and reorganisation of services have considerably reduced the time many patients need to spend in hospital. An increasing number of surgical conditions are now being treated in Day Surgery units. The patient may attend in the morning, have the operation, receive essential aftercare and go home in the afternoon. Procedures undertaken in suitable patients include such things as simple breast operations (e.g. lump removal), hernia repairs, varicose vein treatment, haemorrhoidectomy, vasectomy, circumcision, cataract operations (removing opacities from the lens of the eye). Good communication with the patient and the primary health care team is particularly important. Care after discharge needs special consideration.

The potential advantages of Day Surgery are that postoperative recovery may be better, the risk of infection from hospital is probably lower, the patient spends little time away from home (especially important for children) or work, the management of the surgical workload is more efficient and fewer surgical inpatient beds are required. Day Surgery requires good organisation and management, and special facilities, staffing and training. The number of units in the UK is increasing and it is estimated that within a few years Day Surgery may account overall for about 50 per cent of all surgery, higher in some disciplines and obviously much lower in others.

Surgical treatment of coronary atherosclerosis

The surgical treatment of coronary atherosclerosis relieves the symptoms and improves the outlook for many patients with severe angina pectoris. This involves a major operation in which a fresh arterial blood supply is connected to the coronary artery at a point beyond the blockage caused by the atherosclerotic plaque. Either an artery from the chest wall is joined directly to the coronary artery, or a piece of expendable leg vein (from the patient) is used to plumb a blood supply from the aorta (just above the heart) to the coronary artery.

In some patients a simpler procedure is used – **coronary angioplasty**. This involves passing a special long thin flexible tube through the skin into an artery and then, under X-ray guidance, along the aorta and into the affected coronary vessel. At the end of the tube a small carefully positioned balloon is expanded at the site of the constriction. This compresses the lesion and widens the lumen of the artery. Coronary angioplasty does not involve open surgery and the patient's stay in hospital can be short.

Patients must be very carefully selected and investigated before offering these procedures. There is a small risk of death from coronary surgery but the overall benefit in suitable patients can far outweigh the risks of not having the treatment. These procedures are now commonplace and their use is likely to increase further.

Fracture of the hip

In the UK there are about 40,000 hip fractures every year, and around 200,000 in the US. Most occur in people over 50 years, the majority in women. Osteoporosis is an underlying factor in most cases (see chapter eight, page 193) and many of these fractures are associated with falls in the home. It is estimated that more than a quarter of white women over 60 are likely to suffer a hip fracture.

Fracture of the hip is the common term for a fracture of the **femoral neck**. It involves the upper part of the **femur** (thigh bone) close to the hip joint (see figure 10.1). The head of the femur is the rounded uppermost part. Between this and the long shaft is the short femoral neck. The hip joint consists of the head of the femur and the acetabulum, the cup-like cavity at the side of the pelvis into which the femoral head fits.

Bones have muscles attached to them, pulling in different directions, but normally acting in a co-ordinated and controlled way. After a fracture the muscles tend to pull the bone fragments in unusual directions so that the normal alignment of the bone is lost. In order for the bone ends to reunite without deformity they must be manipulated back into alignment again; this process is known as **reduction** of the fracture. Traction (a steady pull) from systems of weights and pulleys,

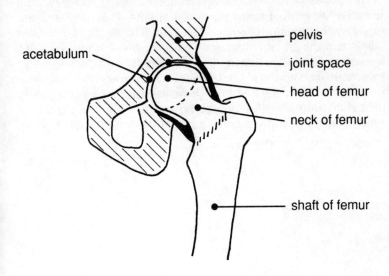

Figure 10.1 The hip joint and upper part of the femur

and splints and plaster casts are used to maintain alignment after reduction and to prevent movement at the fracture site. Hip fractures take several weeks to heal sufficiently to allow weight-bearing without support. In the very elderly such long periods of immobilisation sometimes cause serious, and not infrequently fatal, complications. An alternative is to operate as soon as possible and fix and stabilise the fracture with mechanical devices such as special screws, plates and nails, which are left permanently in position. The type of device used depends on the type of fracture and its anatomical position. Sometimes it is preferable to remove the top of the femur and create a new hip joint using a **prosthesis** (an artificial replacement part). The advantage of these procedures is that the patient can be gently mobilised and out of bed within a day or two.

The management of hip fracture in the elderly with osteoporosis is difficult and the choice of procedure is often far from straightforward. Immobilisation can be hazardous in these patients, yet so can the complications of major surgery and general anaesthesia. Furthermore, internal fixation and prostheses are not always successful and they can give rise to local complications, which sometimes require further surgery. The expected life span of many of these patients is already compromised by the presence of other diseases. The death rate within a few months of hip fracture is higher in the elderly with dementia. The assessment of risk, benefit and the effect of treatment on quality of life as well as on predicted length of life is particularly pertinent in these patients, and particularly difficult. There is still a lack of consensus on some aspects of the treatment of hip fracture in the elderly, and practices can vary between centres.

INDEX